QUICK LOOK SERIES in Veterinary Medicine

CRITICAL CARE

Edited by

Robert J. Murtaugh, DVM, MS

Medical Director
VCA South Shore Animal Hospital
South Weymouth, Massachusetts

Associate Editors

Nishi Dhupa, BVM, MRCVS
James N. Ross, DVM, PhD
Elizabeth Rozanski, DVM
John Rush, DVM, MS

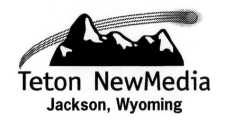

Teton NewMedia
Jackson, Wyoming

Executive Editor: Carroll C. Cann
Development Editor: Susan L. Hunsberger
Editor: Cynthia J. Roantree
Cover Design: Anita Sykes
Typeset by Achorn Graphics, Worcester, MA
Printed by McNaughton & Gunn, Saline, MI
Illustrations by Anne Rains

Teton NewMedia
P.O. Box 4833
4125 South Highway 89, Suite 1
Jackson, WY 83001
1-888-770-3165
http://www.tetonnm.com

Library of Congress Cataloging-in-Publication Data

Critical care / edited by Robert J. Murtaugh; associate editors, Nishi Dhupa ... [et al.].
      p. ; cm.—(Quick look series in veterinary medicine)
   Includes bibliographical references and index.
   ISBN 1-893441-35-0
   1. Veterinary critical care. I. Murtaugh, Robert J. II. Dhupa, Nishi. III. Series.
   [DNLM: 1. Animal Diseases—therapy. 2. Critical Care. SF 778 C934 2001]
SF778.C75 2001
636.089'6028—dc21

                                                    00-066648

Printed and bound by CPI Group (UK) Ltd, Croydon, CR0 4YY

Dedication

Our ability as doctors to practice veterinary critical care medicine is dependent on the skill, knowledge, fortitude, and perseverance of those individuals that pride themselves on being veterinary critical care technicians. A special salute to Donna, Dee, and Valerie for being the leaders in their profession at Tufts University School of Veterinary Medicine.

Preface

It has been ten years since a textbook on veterinary emergency and critical care medicine by a couple of guys named Kaplan and Murtaugh was published (I promised myself I would never do it again!). The world of veterinary emergency and critical care medicine has moved forward by leaps and bounds since that time. In 1992, we had our first resident in veterinary emergency and critical care medicine at Tufts—Dr. Robin Wall finishing her program. Today, there are over 90 residents in many different academic and private practice locations currently training to be specialists in the field. Drs. Rush, Rozanski, Dhupa, Ross, and myself have had the good fortune to be able to influence the training of many past and present residents, now leaders in veterinary emergency and critical care medicine. Additionally, the establishment of student chapters of the Veterinary Emergency and Critical Care Society on most veterinary campuses, the certification of veterinary technicians in the specialty of veterinary emergency and critical care medicine, the insertion of classroom and rotational training in the Specialty for many students of veterinary medicine, and the blossoming of ICU units at a multitude of veterinary colleges and schools speaks to the increasing prominence and importance of veterinary emergency and critical care medicine. With that backdrop, I can state unequivocally that it was especially rewarding to write this textbook in concert with the entire recent cast of faculty and residents from Tufts University School of Veterinary Medicine. We hope you will find this text a useful tool in your study and practice of critical care medicine.

Robert Murtaugh

Table of Contents

Contributors

Lilian Cornejo, DVM
Tufts University
School of Veterinary Medicine
North Grafton, Massachusetts

Armelle DeLaforcade, DVM
Tufts University
School of Veterinary Medicine
North Grafton, Massachusetts

Nishi Dhupa, BVM, MRCVS
Cornell University
College of Veterinary Medicine
Ithaca, New York

Alison Gaynor, DVM, DACVIM, DACVECC
North Grafton, Massachusetts

Andrea Gilbert, DVM
Bolton, Massachusetts

Daniel Hecht, DVM
Animal Emergency Center
West Bridgewater, Massachusetts

Justine Johnson, DVM
Ocean States Veterinary Referral Center
Warwick, Rhode Island

Ari Jutkowitz, DVM
Tufts University
School of Veterinary Medicine
North Grafton, Massachusetts

Ann Marie Manning, DVM
Angell Memorial Animal Hospital
Boston, Massachusetts

Maureen McMichael, DVM
Texas A&M University
College of Veterinary Medicine
College Station, Texas

Steven Mensack, DVM
Private Practice
Detroit, Michigan

Kari Moore, DVM
BCA Veterinary Referral Associates
Gaithersburg, Maryland

Erika Zsombor-Murray, DVM
Dove Lewis Emergency Animal Hospital
Portland, Oregon

Robert J. Murtaugh, DVM, MS
VCA South Shore Animal Hospital
South Weymouth, Massachusetts

Theresa O'Toole, DVM
Tufts University
School of Veterinary Medicine
North Grafton, Massachusetts

Lisa Powell, DVM
Department of Small Animal Clinical Sciences
College of Veterinary Medicine
University of Minnesota
St. Paul, Minnesota

Jeffrey Proulx, DVM
Society for Prevention of Cruelty to Animals
San Francisco, California

James N. Ross, DVM, PhD
Department of Clinical Sciences
Tufts University
School of Veterinary Medicine
North Grafton, Massachusetts

Elizabeth Rozanski, DVM
Assistant Professor
Emergency Critical Care
Department of Clinical Sciences
Tufts University
School of Veterinary Medicine
North Grafton, Massachusetts

John Rush, DVM
Associate Professor
Head, Section of Emergency Critical Care
Department of Clinical Sciences
Tufts University
School of Veterinary Medicine
North Grafton, Massachusetts

Nancy Taylor, DVM
Puget Sound Veterinary Pavillion
Tacoma, Washington

QUICK LOOK SERIES IN VETERINARY MEDICINE
CRITICAL CARE

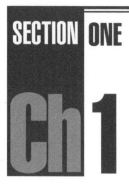
Sodium Chloride Balance

Erika Zsombor-Murray

A   Body Fluid Components

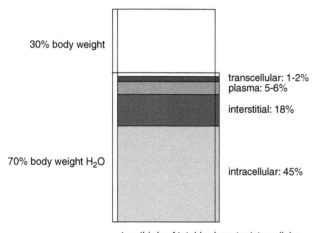

30% body weight

transcellular: 1-2%
plasma: 5-6%

interstitial: 18%

70% body weight H_2O

intracellular: 45%

- two-thirds of total-body water intracellular

extracellular: 80% interstitial fluid
                   20% plasma

B   Gastrointestinal Absorption of Sodium

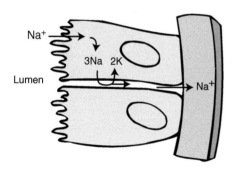

Na^+

Lumen

3Na 2K

Na^+

C

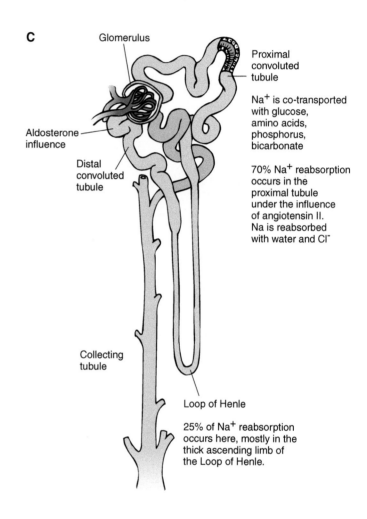

Glomerulus

Proximal convoluted tubule

Na^+ is co-transported with glucose, amino acids, phosphorus, bicarbonate

Aldosterone influence

70% Na^+ reabsorption occurs in the proximal tubule under the influence of angiotensin II. Na is reabsorbed with water and Cl^-

Distal convoluted tubule

Collecting tubule

Loop of Henle

25% of Na^+ reabsorption occurs here, mostly in the thick ascending limb of the Loop of Henle.

D   Angiotensin II and Sodium Reabsorption

1. directly increases sodium reabsorption by the tubular epithelial cells of the proximal convoluted tubule;
2. causes increased aldosterone secretion from the adrenal cortex;
3. causes constriction of the efferent renal arteriole and dilation of the afferent renal arteriole, which acts to improve the glomerular filtration rate (GFR).

Sodium is the principle cation of the extracellular fluid (ECF). Its presence, in appropriate concentrations, is vital for the maintenance of osmolality within the ECF (**Part A**). Combined with the principle extracellular anions (chloride and bicarbonate), sodium provides close to 95% of the osmolarly active solutes within the ECF. Serum osmolality can be estimated by using the following equation:

$$2Na(mEq/L) + BUN(mg/dL)/2.8 + Glucose(mg/dL)/18$$

The normal range for serum osmolality is 290–310 mOsm/kg in dogs and 290–330 mOsm/kg in cats. There should not be more than a 10 mOsm/kg difference between the calculated and measured serum osmolality. An increased osmolar gap signifies that measured sodium values are artificially low owing to laboratory error from hyperlipidemia or hyperproteinemia or that unmeasured solute, such as mannitol or ethylene glycol metabolites, is present in the serum.

Serum osmolality is controlled tightly in an effort to prevent adverse changes in the water balance between the extracellular and intracellular fluid (ICF) compartments. Water movement is dependent on changes in the concentration of molecules which cannot readily cross cell membranes. The tonicity or effective osmolality of the ECF and ICF reflects the concentration of these osmotically-active molecules (e.g., glucose, sodium). Osmoles permeable to cell membranes (e.g., urea), distribute equally between the 2 body fluid compartments. Increases in urea concentration do not affect water balance or tonicity. Changes in sodium concentration will affect both tonicity and osmolality. Tonicity can be estimated using the following formula:

$$2Na(mEq/L) + Glucose(mg/dL)/18$$

Regulation of Osmolality

Mechanoreceptors within the cardiac atria, high-pressure receptors in the carotid arteries, and the juxtaglomerular apparatus within the kidneys sense effective circulating volume. If it is perceived that this ECF volume is low, the kidneys act to retain sodium and water. Glomerulotubular balance, aldosterone, atrial natriuretic peptide (ANP), and renal hemodynamic factors mediate sodium excretion or retention.

GI Sodium and Chloride Absorption

Sodium and chloride are absorbed in the GI tract. A total of 25–30 gm of sodium are absorbed daily from the small intestine, 80% of which is derived from digestive secretions. Sodium passively diffuses down its concentration gradient from the lumen (Na = 142 mEq/L), across the brush border, and into the cytosol of the gut epithelial cells (Na = 50 mEq/L). The low intracellular sodium concentration is maintained by the sodium-potassium ATPase pumps (Na^+, K^+ ATPase pumps), located in the basolateral walls of the gut epithelial cells. Sodium is pumped into the intercellular spaces, and chloride passively follows sodium to maintain electroneurality (**Part B**). Water follows the osmotic gradient created by this large concentration of ions within the intercellular space. In the dehydrated state, increased concentration of aldosterone is secreted, and acts to enhance sodium reabsorption by the intestinal epithelial cells. This effect is especially pronounced in the colon where almost all water and sodium chloride are absorbed from fecal material. The epithelium of the ileum and colon has an exchange protein, which allows secretion of bicarbonate into the lumen in exchange for the absorption of chloride. Chloride moves by facilitated diffusion through the basolateral cell membrane and into the intercellular space.

Sodium Reabsorption

Sodium and chloride are freely filtered by the glomerulus, and the kidneys reabsorb 99.5% of filtered sodium (**Part C**). The energy driving sodium reabsorption within the kidneys derives from the chemical and electrical gradients created by the Na, K-ATPase pumps. Low intracellular sodium concentration allows sodium to passively diffuse into the tubular cells and then to be actively pumped out the basolateral membrane.

In the early proximal tubule, sodium is co-transported with glucose, amino acids, phosphate, and bicarbonate, while in the latter portion of the proximal tubule, sodium is reabsorbed primarily with chloride. This cumulative reabsorption of ions creates an osmotic difference across the cell membranes, and water is reabsorbed along with sodium.

Most of the sodium reabsorption occurs in the thick ascending limb of the loop of Henle. A smaller proportion of sodium is absorbed passively in the thin descending and ascending limbs. Sodium is actively transported in the thick ascending limb, but unlike other portions of the nephron, the tubular epithelium here is impermeable to water.

Sodium and chloride reabsorption in the distal convoluted tubule is accomplished in the same manner as in the proximal convoluted tubule. The collecting tubule reabsorbs 5% of filtered sodium. Aldosterone concentration determines the precise amount reabsorbed in these locations.

Regulation of Sodium Reabsorption

Decreased perfusion of the macula densa from hypotension or from a decrease in effective circulating volume is interpreted as hyponatremia and hypochloremia. The macula densa then stimulates the juxta glomerular cells to release renin. Renin cleaves angiotensinogen to angiotensin I, which is then converted to angiotensin II in the lungs. Renin release also occurs in response to beta-1 adrenergic stimulation, initiated by the baroreceptors of the atria, carotid sinus, and aortic arch. Angiotensin II acts in 3 ways to increase sodium reabsorption (**Part D**).

Aldosterone acts on the distal convoluted tubule to enhance sodium reabsorption by opening and increasing the number of luminal sodium channels. Prolonged exposure to aldosterone increases the activity and density of the Na,K-ATPase pumps located in the basolateral membrane. Increased levels of aldosterone are secreted in response to hyperkalemia, angiotensin II, and a decrease in dietary sodium intake. Aldosterone levels are diminished when there is an increase in dietary sodium intake and elevated plasma concentration of ANP.

The sympathetic nervous system (SNS) directly and indirectly (renin release) affects sodium reabsorption. Direct effects of the SNS on sodium reabsorption are mediated by changes in renal hemodynamic factors and through redistribution of renal blood flow from the cortical to the juxtamedullary nephrons. Cortical nephrons have shorter loops of Henle and thus are less effective at sodium reabsorption compared to the juxtamedullary nephrons.

Atrial natriuretic peptide (ANP) is produced primarily within the atrial myocytes and is released into circulation when the cardiac atria become distended. Its effects include relaxation of the vascular smooth muscle, decreased production of angiotensin II and aldosterone, and decreasing sodium reabsorption in the collecting tubule.

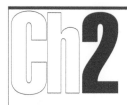

Hypernatremia and Hyponatremia

Erika Zsombor-Murray

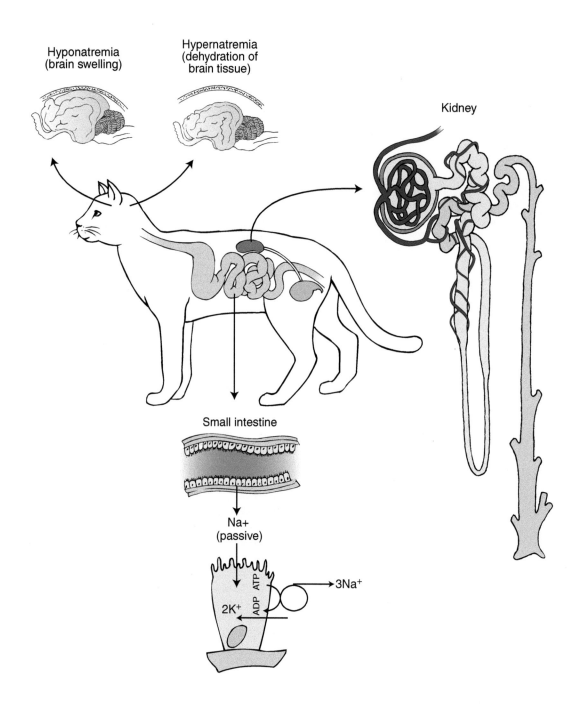

Causes of Hypernatremia

Sodium concentrations greater than 155 mEq/L are termed hypernatremia (**Figure**). This occurs when pure water is lost in excess of sodium but also can be induced when sodium-containing fluids are administered. Pure water loss occurs in patients with central or nephrogenic diabetes insipidus who are denied access to water; with osmotic diuresis with mannitol or glucose; with hyperventilation; with extensive burns; when there is a lack of water intake from withholding water; with hypothalamic disease causing decreased thirst; and rarely from hyperaldosteronism. Iatrogenic causes of hypernatremia include the administration of hypertonic saline solution (IV or via enema) and IV administration of sodium bicarbonate in significant quantities.

Clinical Signs of Hypernatremia

When sodium concentrations exceed 170 mEq/L, intracellular dehydration results, and since brain cells are particularly sensitive to dehydration, neurological signs are observed. Patients exhibit lethargy and weakness in the early stages. If untreated, the clinical signs will progress to seizures, coma, and death. In general, the severity of the clinical signs appears to be more dependent on the rapidity of the sodium concentration change, rather than on the degree of hypernatremia.

Treatment of Hypernatremia

If the hypernatremia is chronic and has evolved over several days, sodium concentration needs to be reduced gradually to normal levels through the administration of IV fluids. By the first 3 to 5 days of hypernatremia, brain cells have synthesized intracellular idiogenic osmoles to help prevent further dehydration of the neurons. If hypernatremia is corrected too rapidly, the idiogenic osmoles cannot be eliminated quickly enough and will draw water into the neurons, resulting in the development of edema in the central nervous system (CNS). In chronic hypernatremia, the amount of free water required to eliminate the deficit should be administered over 48 to 72 hours, so that sodium concentrations fall at a rate of less than 1 mEq/hr. The free water deficit can be estimated using the following formula:

0.6 × body weight (kg) × (1 − 140/serum Na)
= L of free water required

1 L of 5% dextrose in water (D5W)
= 1 L of free water

1 L of 0.45% saline + 2.5% dextrose in water
= 0.5 L of free water

If hypernatremic patients are exhibiting neurological signs, if the sodium concentration is greater than 170 mEq/L, or if the hypernatremia has persisted for 3 days, 0.45% or 0.9% saline solution should be used for the initial corrective treatment, instead of D5W. This approach minimizes the potential for too rapid a decrease in plasma sodium concentration. Regardless of the crystalloid fluid chosen or the rate of IV fluid administration, hypernatremic patients need frequent and serial monitoring and reassessment. Fluid therapy should be adjusted and individualized to best meet the patient's requirements, and the clinician must address treatment (e.g., antidiuretic hormone administration) to the underlying disease process, to maintain serum sodium concentration corrected with fluid therapy.

Causes of Hyponatremia

Normally when sodium is lost, the body reacts by decreasing ADH release, causing urine to become more dilute and thereby returning plasma osmolality to normal (see **Figure**). If there is significant volume depletion accompanying hyponatremia, this down-regulation of ADH secretion is overridden and ADH secretion is enhanced. Free water is reabsorbed and hyponatremia is potentiated. Most cases of hypoadrenocorticism are due in part to aldosterone deficiency. This allows sodium loss, volume depletion, ADH release, and thirst, resulting in hyponatremia. In polyuric renal failure, vomiting causes loss of both sodium and water, polyuria enhances volume depletion, and ADH release is stimulated. This can result in hyponatremia. Inappropriate ADH secretion is rare in dogs but can occur with dirofilariasis, hypothalamic disease, or drug therapy (barbiturates, vincristine, cyclophosphamide, narcotics, chloramphenicol).

Clinical Signs of Hyponatremia

The accompanying hypo-osmolality of plasma associated with the development of hyponatremia causes water to move intracellularly. The clinical signs of hyponatremia are due to the resultant cerebral edema and include depression, lethargy, seizures, and coma. As with hypernatremia, clinical signs are seen more often when hyponatremia develops rapidly, rather than when it is severe. The most severe complications of hyponatremia are seen when sodium concentration drops at a rate of >0.5 mEq/L/hr, or when serum sodium concentration is <120 mEq/L. Clinical signs are often absent in patients with chronic hyponatremia because the CNS has had time to adjust to plasma hypotonicity.

Treatment for Hyponatremia

Correction of hyponatremia involves identifying and correcting the underlying cause, and improving serum sodium concentration and serum osmolality if clinically necessary. Aggressive and rapid correction of chronic hyponatremia can be more deleterious to patients than the electrolyte imbalance itself. Osmotic demyelination syndrome develops 3 to 4 days after too rapid correction of chronic hyponatremia. Patients with this syndrome develop weakness, lethargy, ataxia and progress to hypermetria and quadriparesis. Chronically hyponatremic patients who are normovolemic often are treated most easily with fluid restriction. During the period of fluid restriction, it is important to carefully monitor the patient's neurological and cardiovascular status. Acutely hyponatremic patients exhibiting neurological signs should be treated with IV administration of LRS or normal saline solution. The IV fluid rate should be set to increase serum sodium concentration, but at a rate of less than 10 to 12 mEq/L/day (0.5 mEq/L/hr). The sodium deficit can be calculated using the following formula:

(Normal serum Na − measured serum Na)
× 0.6 × (Body weight in kg) = Required mEq of Na

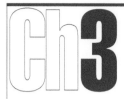

Potassium Homeostasis and Hypokalemia

Nancy S. Taylor

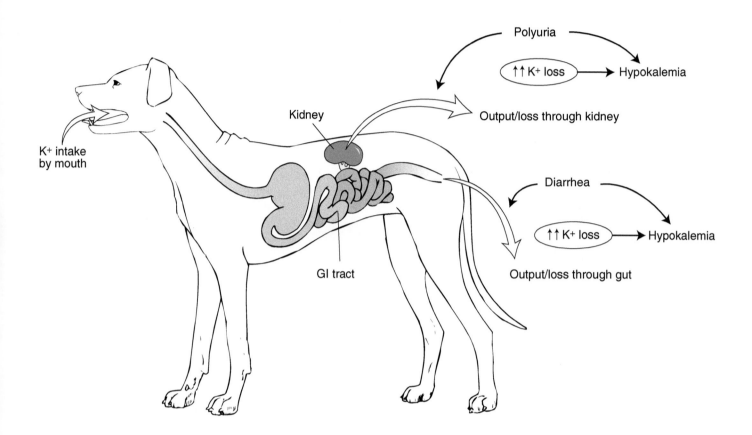

Treatment of Hypokalemia	
Serum [K+]	[K+] / liter of IV fluids
3.0 - 3.5 meq/L	30 meq/L
2.5 - 3.0 meq/L	40 meq/L
2.0 - 2.5 meq/L	50 meq/L
<2.0 meq/L	60 meq/L

Maximal infusion rate for K+ = 0.5 meq/kg/hour

Clinical Signs with Hypokalemia
1. Muscle weakness
2. Cardiac conduction abnormalities
3. Limited drug effectiveness

Potassium derangements often occur in critical patients and may be life threatening. Therefore an understanding of potassium homeostasis and treatment of any abnormalities is crucial for the outcome of the critically ill animal.

Potassium is the most abundant cation found in the mammalian body and has many important roles for maintenance of normal cell function. The most important function of potassium is its role in generating the resting cell membrane potential. Intracellular potassium is also important in enzyme systems that are responsible for cell growth through DNA, glycogen, and protein synthesis. Potassium is a key player in neuromuscular transmission and abnormalities in potassium homeostasis can lead to cardiac and skeletal muscle dysfunctions.

Normal Homeostasis

Most potassium is intracellular (95–98%) while the remaining (2–5%) is extracellular. Extracellular potassium is tightly regulated to optimize cardiac and skeletal muscle function. In cats and dogs, serum potassium concentration is maintained between 3.5 and 5.5mEq/L.

The regulation of potassium involves a balance between intake, excretion, and distribution within the body. Potassium is ingested in the diet and absorbed through the gastrointestinal tract. Most of the potassium derived from the diet, as well as from cellular breakdown, is removed by the kidneys (90–95%). A small amount (5–10%) is excreted in the stool.

Generally, a load of potassium ingested through the diet is dealt with immediately by translocation of potassium from the extracellular to the intracellular fluids, and then through renal excretion over the following two days. Insulin and catecholamines (through action on β_2-adrenergic receptors) will enhance uptake of potassium by the liver and muscles in response to an acute potassium load. The colon and kidneys can also increase their excretion of potassium. Increased potassium concentrations, aldosterone release, and increased distal renal tubular flow rates will all contribute to enhanced renal excretion of potassium.

Metabolic acidosis, due to an increase in the serum hydrogen ion concentration will cause potassium to move out of cells in exchange for excess hydrogen ion while metabolic alkalosis will cause potassium to redistribute into cells. This hydrogen/potassium exchange mechanism aids in keeping the pH of the blood in a normal range.

Hypokalemia

Hypokalemia can result from inadequate intake, increased excretion through polyuria or diarrhea, or from intracellular translocation of potassium. Lack of adequate intake alone rarely causes hypokalemia unless it occurs in combination with increased gastrointestinal or renal loss. The most common causes for hypokalemia are anorexia, vomiting, chronic renal failure, and diuretic therapy. Cats with feline urologic syndrome often develop hypokalemia during postobstructive diuresis. Deficits due to translocation can be a result of alkalosis, insulin administration, and hyperthyroidism. Epinephrine release associated with the stress of illness can also contribute to hypokalemia. Hypokalemia can also be seen in hyperadrenocorticism due to the mineralcorticoid effects of excess endogenous steroids.

Most critically ill patients on limited oral intake and intravenous fluid therapy develop hypokalemia, and require potassium supplementation.

Clinical Signs

The clinical signs associated with decreased serum potassium are most often a result of effects on cardiac or skeletal muscle and the kidney. The patient may have subtle clinical signs or obvious muscle weakness. Weakness associated with hypokalemia may manifest as ventroflexion of the neck or a stiff stilted gait. Muscle weakness is usually seen when serum potassium levels fall below 3.0 mEq/L. If the serum potassium level falls below 2.5 mEq/L, serum creatine kinase activity will elevate. Severe rhabdomyolysis may occur at levels below 2.0 mEq/L.

In the presence of hypokalemia the resting membrane potential of a cell becomes more negative which creates a larger difference between the resting and threshold membrane potential. This results in decreased excitability, prolonged repolarization, and increased automaticity of the muscle cells. Electrocardiographic manifestations may include ST-segment depression and reduced amplitude of T-waves. Prolonged QT intervals and various ventricular and supraventricular arrhythmias may develop as a result of hypokalemia.

Hypokalemia can also cause the myocardium to be refractory to the effects of Class I antiarrhythmic agents (lidocaine, quinidine, and procainamide) and potassium levels should be measured and corrected in dogs with ventricular arrhythmias unresponsive to antiarrhythmic therapy.

Commonly, hypokalemia occurs with metabolic alkalosis due to enhanced renal excretion of potassium. Weight loss, poor hair coat, decreased muscle mass, and delayed growth can also occur in chronic hypokalemic states. This is a result of the effects of potassium on cell growth.

Treatment

In situations of mild hypokalemia, oral supplementation with potassium gluconate (Tumil-K, Daniels Pharmaceuticals) may be all that is required. Dogs require 2–4 mEq of potassium per day depending on the size of the dog. Cats require potassium gluconate at 2.5–5 mEq per day divided into two or three doses, depending on the severity of hypokalemia and size of the cat. The signs of muscle weakness usually resolve in 7–14 days after initiating treatment.

Maintenance of potassium supplementation is recommended at a dosage of 1–2 mEq/day until the underlying cause of the hypokalemia has been determined and corrected. Many cats in renal failure require long-long therapy of potassium at a dosage of 2–4 mEq/day. The dosage should be determined by monitoring serum potassium levels and the clinical response to treatment.

Animals that are anorexic or vomiting and those with moderate to severe hypokalemia (<2.5 mEq/L) may require intravenous supplementation of potassium. Potassium chloride is usually chosen for intravenous use. Potassium supplementation is usually based on clinical signs and serum values (**Figure**). Potassium should not be administered faster than 0.5 mEq/kg/hour and never administered as a straight bolus. Fatal cardiac bradyarrhythmias can occur with overzealous supplementation. It is recommended that fluids with potassium supplementation be administered through fluid infusion pumps in order to prevent iatrogenic hyperkalemia and possible death. Concentrations of greater than 60 mEq/L should be avoided as these concentrations may cause pain and sclerosis at the intravenous catheter site.

There may be an initial decrease in serum potassium levels with the onset of intravenous potassium supplementation as a result of dilutional effects, increased renal tubular flow, and cellular uptake of potassium, especially in fluids containing glucose. Concomitant administration of sodium bicarbonate will also promote uptake of potassium into the cells and should be used with caution.

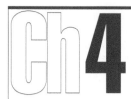

Hyperkalemia

Nancy S. Taylor

A Causes of Hyperkalemia

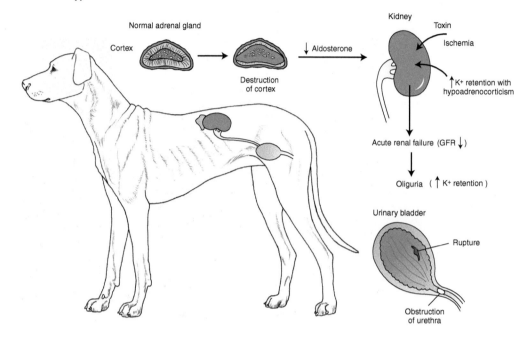

B

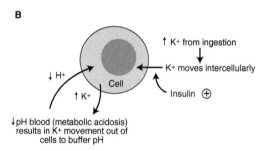

C ECG Manifestations of Hyperkalemia

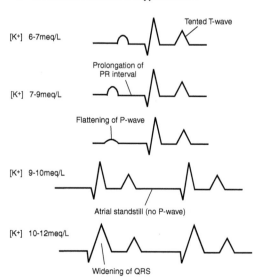

D Treatment

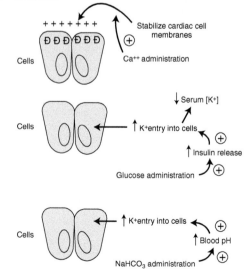

Hyperkalemia is uncommon in the presence of normal renal function. It can result from excessive intake, inadequate excretion, or shifting of potassium from cells into plasma.

Hyperkalemia due to excessive intake is rare because large potassium loads are rapidly translocated into cells and then excreted by the kidneys. Usually hyperkalemia from excessive "intake" is iatrogenic and related to potassium being added to IV fluids in excessive amounts or administered too rapidly. IV potassium administration should not exceed 0.5 mEq/kg/hr.

Inadequate excretion occurs with urethral obstruction, rupture of the urinary bladder or ureters, oliguric or anuric renal failure, hypoadrenocorticism, and some types of GI diseases (whipworm infestation, salmonellosis, and duodenal perforation) (**Part A**).

Translocation of potassium out of cells can cause mild to moderate hyperkalemia (5–7 mEq/L). This is seen with metabolic acidosis as a result of excess hydrogen ions being buffered in cells and potassium being exchanged to maintain electroneutrality (**Part B**).

Patients with diabetes mellitus, with or without ketoacidosis (DKA), may actually be depleted of total potassium but have increased levels of serum potassium due to insulin deficiency and acidosis (with DKA). Insulin activity promotes the cellular uptake of potassium. Additionally, extracellular hyperosmolality due to hyperglycemia will cause increased extraction of water from the cells, thereby increasing the intracellular potassium concentration and exacerbating the shift of potassium from inside the cell to outside the cell. Following IV administration of fluids and insulin therapy, these patients often quickly become hypokalemic.

Pseudohyperkalemia may result from poor venipuncture technique, thrombocytosis, leukocytosis, and in vitro hemolysis of blood in Akitas.

Signs

The clinical signs associated with hyperkalemia are usually a result of changes in the resting membrane potential of cells. The increased extracellular potassium concentration makes the resting membrane potential less negative. This change brings the resting membrane potential and threshold potentials closer together, making the membrane more excitable. This produces a weaker action potential when threshold is reached. With severe hyperkalemia, the resting potential may actually drop below threshold, and the cell then becomes unable to depolarize and is no longer excitable.

ECG manifestations of mild hyperkalemia include the development of high-peaked T waves. Hyperkalemia does not usually prolong the QT interval. This feature is observed with other disorders causing peaked T waves. ECG changes associated with moderate to severe hyperkalemia include prolongation of the PR interval as seen with cardiopulmonary arrest (**Part C**).

The effects of hyperkalemia on other muscle cells can result in abdominal pain, diarrhea, and flaccid paralysis of the limbs. In severe cases, respiratory paralysis may be seen.

Treatment

Moderate hyperkalemia (6.0–8.0 mEq/L) usually does not cause life-threatening cardiac arrhythmias, and treatment includes IV administration of potassium-free fluids as well as elimination of the factors causing the hyperkalemia.

In situations where serum potassium levels exceed 8.0 mEq/L, or where cardiotoxicity is seen, initiation of further treatment is required. Options include the IV administration of calcium gluconate, sodium bicarbonate, and/or insulin/dextrose (**Part D**).

Calcium will antagonize the cardiac effects of hyperkalemia without altering the plasma concentration of potassium. Calcium gluconate 10% can be administered IV at a dose of 50–100 mg/kg over 10–20 minutes, while monitoring the patient's ECG. If bradycardia develops, calcium administration should be stopped. The effects of calcium usually last <1 hour, and further treatments are necessary to lower the serum potassium level. Calcium gluconate treatment generally is reserved for severe life-threatening cardiotoxicity from hyperkalemia (e.g., severe pre–cardiac arrest bradycardia).

Infusions of hypertonic glucose solutions will cause potassium to be shifted back into the cells through the effects associated with increased endogenous insulin secretion. Insulin moves both glucose and potassium into the cells. Twenty percent glucose can be administered as an IV bolus (0.5–1.0 gm/kg). Regular insulin (0.5 IU/kg) can be co-administered as an IV bolus concurrently with the dextrose. Blood glucose levels need to be monitored to prevent hypoglycemia. IV fluids must be supplemented with dextrose at 2.5%–5.0% following glucose/insulin bolus administration. The use of glucose alone will lower the potassium level within 1 hour, with effects lasting several hours. The addition of insulin will cause a more immediate effect, and is used in patients with severe hyperkalemia.

Sodium bicarbonate also will help lower serum potassium levels by causing potassium to shift into the cells, in exchange for hydrogen ion, which moves into the extracellular space. Administration of sodium bicarbonate will lower the potassium concentration within minutes to 1 hour, and this effect lasts several hours. If the patient has metabolic acidosis, the dose administered is based on the calculated base deficit (Measured base deficit × Weight in kg × 0.3). One-third of this calculated dose is administered rapidly by the IV route, and repeat administration is dependent on reassessment of the base deficit and serum potassium levels. In nonacidotic patients, sodium bicarbonate can still be given to reduce serum potassium levels. An empiric dose of 0.5–1.0 mEq/kg administered IV over 10–15 minutes is recommended followed by re-evaluation of the patient's ECG and serum potassium concentration.

Sodium bicarbonate administration needs to be used judiciously in cardiac and oliguric renal failure patients, as fluid overload could occur with excessive administration of sodium. Similarly, sodium bicarbonate should be used with caution in hypocalcemic animals because sodium bicarbonate administration can reduce plasma ionized calcium levels. As cats with urethral obstruction may have an ionized hypocalcemia, treatment of glucose and insulin may be preferred over the use of sodium bicarbonate, except in cases with severe metabolic acidosis.

Conclusion

Management of serum potassium levels is imperative in critically ill patients. Hyperkalemia can result in deadly arrhythmias if not treated appropriately.

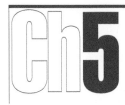

Fluid Therapy I: Crystalloids

Erika Zsombor-Murray

A   IV Route

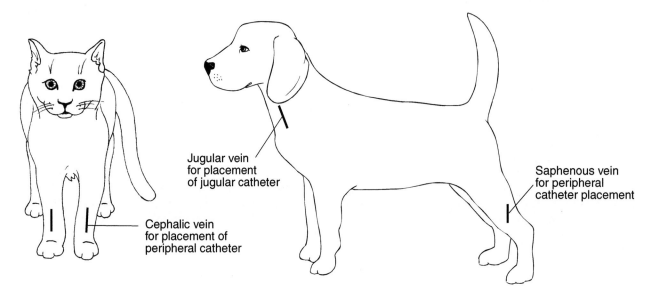

Jugular vein
for placement
of jugular catheter

Cephalic vein
for placement of
peripheral catheter

Saphenous vein
for peripheral
catheter placement

B   Placement of Intraosseus Catheters

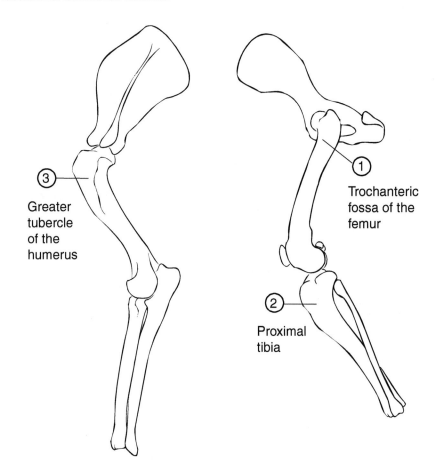

③ Greater
tubercle
of the
humerus

① Trochanteric
fossa of the
femur

② Proximal
tibia

Fluid therapy is one of the most widely used treatments in veterinary medicine. Despite familiarity with the use of fluids, the veterinarian should carefully assess every patient to determine the optimum fluid type, volume, route, and rate of administration. There are many options regarding fluid choice. For some conditions, such as shock, restoring tissue with adequate fluid volume is more critical than the type of crystalloid fluid chosen. In most other cases, it is helpful to guide IV fluid choice through knowledge of a patient's hemodynamic status, serum electrolyte measurements, acid-base balance, and suspected or confirmed underlying disease. This chapter focuses on the administration of crystalloid solutions.

Indications for IV Crystalloid Fluid Therapy

Crystalloid solutions consist predominantly of water, with sodium chloride or glucose as the primary component. The concentrations of electrolytes (sodium, chloride, potassium, magnesium, and calcium), glucose, and bicarbonate precursors (lactate, acetate) vary between solutions. Along with the pH and osmolality of the solutions, these factors help to determine which fluid is the most appropriate choice in any given situation. IV crystalloid fluid administration should be part of the therapeutic plan in the following circumstances:

1. Severe dehydration, hypovolemia, and non-cardiogenic shock, where expansion of the intravascular volume to normal or supranormal levels is necessary to establish adequate tissue perfusion and oxygen delivery.
2. Correction of electrolyte imbalances and restoration of acid-base balance to normal.
3. With IV constant rate infusions (CRIs) for drug administration. For example, diabetic ketoacidotic (DKA) patients are dehydrated at presentation, and regular insulin given by intramuscular or subcutaneous injections may be variably absorbed. A CRI of regular insulin ensures a continuous and even supply of insulin to the tissues. Other drugs commonly administered by means of a CRI include antiarrhythmic agents (lidocaine, procainamide), pressor agents (dopamine, dobutamine), vasodilators (nitroprusside), electrolytes (calcium gluconate, potassium phosphate), anesthetics (pentobarbitol, propofol), neuromuscular blockers (atracurium), and antiemetics (metoclopromide).
4. During surgical procedures, intraoperative IV fluid administration improves the safety of general anesthesia, helps to maintain intravascular volume and systemic arterial blood pressure, and provides for vascular access in case of unforeseen emergency (e.g. bradycardia, cardiopulmonary arrest).
5. As the mainstay of treatment of many medical diseases including renal insufficiency or failure, pancreatitis, GI disease with vomiting, addisonian crisis, sepsis, and DKA.

Routes of Crystalloid Fluid Administration

Crystalloid fluid therapy can be administered by the enteral, subcutaneous, IV, intraosseous, and intraperitoneal routes. Each method of delivery has advantages and disadvantages.

Enteral Route

The oral route is the most physiologic and can be used to rehydrate a mild to moderately dehydrated patient that is not vomiting and that has good control of the airway. Using this route in patients with esophageal or neurological disease can result in aspiration pneumonia. This route of administration is ineffective for achieving rapid clinical benefit. Enteral feeding tubes can be used to facilitate the administration of isotonic, balanced, electrolyte- and glucose-containing solutions.

Subcutaneous Route

Administering fluids subcutaneously should be reserved for the mildly dehydrated patient. Patients with shock or moderate to severe dehydration will not benefit from the subcutaneous administration of fluids. The volume of fluid required should be estimated. The volume delivered with each administration will depend on patient comfort, and no more than 10–20 mls/kg should be administered to any one site. Only fluids without dextrose (e.g. LRS, 0.9% saline) should be administered subcutaneously, and this route should not be used in patient's whose skin appears infected or diseased.

IV Route

In any seriously ill patient, the IV route is preferred for administering fluids. Moderately to severely dehydrated patients and shock victims require IV crystalloid fluid therapy. This route provides for rapid and effective expansion of the intravascular volume. Catheters can be placed in the cephalic, saphenous, and jugular veins (**Part A**). If peripheral vasoconstriction frustrates attempts to place percutaneous IV catheters, venous cutdowns should be attempted to gain venous access.

Intraosseous Route

This route is often useful in pediatric patients, birds, and other small exotics as well as initially for animals in shock in which the peripheral veins are small and collapsed. Sterile technique is needed to place a bone marrow needle or hypodermic needle into the proximal tibia, trochanteric fossa of the femur, or the greater tubercle of the humerus (**Part B**). In birds, the distal end of the ulna is a common site, as all pneumatic bones must be avoided.

Intraperitoneal Route

This route should be used only if the IV and intraosseous routes are inaccessible, and should be considered as a stopgap measure to improve vascular volume until the IV or intraosseous routes become accessible. Sterile technique is used to prepare a site between the umbilicus and the pubic bone. A 16 to 22 gauge hypodermic needle or catheter is used to gain access to the peritoneum and a calculated dose of an isotonic, balanced electrolyte solution is administered. The use of dextrose in the solution is discouraged as the presence of dextrose will raise the osmolality of the balanced electrolyte solution and will draw water from the vascular, interstitial, and intracellular spaces, possibly worsening the patient's hydration. This route should never be used in any patient suspected of having a septic peritonitis or about to undergo abdominal exploratory surgery.

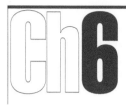

Fluid Therapy II: Crystalloids

Erika Zsombor-Murray

	Ringer's solution	LRS	Plasmalyte A	Normosol- R	0.9% Saline	0.45% Saline	5% Dextrose in water	Normosol- M	Plasmalyte 56	Plasmalyte M
Osmolality (mOsm/L)	312	274	296	296	308	154	278	406	112	406
pH	5.5	6.5	7.4	6.0	5.5	–	5.0	6.0		
Calories (kcal/L)	–	9	18	18	–	–	170			
Na (mEq/L)	147	130	140	140	154	77	–	40	40	40
K (mEq/L)	4	4	5	5	–	–	–	16	13	16
Cl (mEq/L)	156	109	98	98	154	77	–	40	40	40
Ca (mEq/L)	5	3	–	–	–	–	–	5	–	5
Mg (mEq/L)	–	–	3	3	–	–	–	3	3	3
Bicarbonate precurser (mEq/L)	–	28 lactate	27 acetate	27 acetate	–	–	–	16 acetate	16 acetate	12 acetate
Dextrose (gm/L)	–	–	–	–	–	–	50	50	–	50

Volume and Rate of IV Fluid Administration

IV crystalloid fluids are used most often to correct dehydration and for initial resuscitation of a patient in shock. In shock, the goal is to correct or improve tissue perfusion to normal as quickly as possible. For dogs in shock, the dose of crystalloid solution is generally 60–90 ml/kg, and for cats it is generally 40–60 ml/kg. One third to one half of this calculated volume is administered over 10 to 20 minutes, and the patient is reassessed continually by evaluation of heart rate, mucous membrane color, pulse quality, blood pressure, and mentation. If shock is ongoing, the remainder of the calculated resuscitation volume (and more if needed) is administered. If crystalloid administration is not sufficient to reverse shock or sustain resuscitation, colloid administration may be indicated (see Chapter 13). Studies in healthy subjects reveal that one-third of the crystalloid fluid volume remains in the intravascular space 1 hour after infusion, whereas two-thirds is distributed to the interstitium. While this is beneficial in dehydrated patients and adequate for the resuscitation of many shock victims, septic shock patients and some hypovolemic shock patients will require IV colloid fluid therapy for stabilization. In critical patients with decreased colloid osmotic pressure, only 20% of the crystalloid fluid volume administered stays within the vasculature at 60 minutes, and the entire crystalloid fluid volume is in the interstitium by 100 minutes. The increased interstitial volume does little to improve circulatory function and often worsens oxygen transport to the tissues. Such patients require colloid therapy in addition to crystalloid fluid therapy.

For dehydration, the goal is to correct the fluid volume deficit over 24–48 hours. The estimated volume needed is calculated by estimating and adding (1) dehydration volume, (2) maintenance volume (urine, fecal, and respiratory outputs) and, (3) daily ongoing disease-related fluid losses (diarrhea, polyuria, etc).

1. % dehydration × body weight (kg) = ml of fluid e.g. 10% × 10 kg = 1000 ml
2. 40 to 60 ml/kg body weight = maintenance fluid estimate e.g. 60 ml × 10 kg = 600 ml
3. Estimated ongoing, disease-related losses e.g. 500 ml
   Total volume calculated to be infused = 1000 + 600 + 500 = 2100 mL

It is often simplest to divide the total volume to be infused by 24 hours to obtain an hourly rate of fluid administration. Other methods include administering one-third to one-half of the dehydration volume (333 to 500 ml in the example above) over the first 4 hours, and the remaining volume (1600 to 1777 ml) over the last 20 hours. This calculated estimate also can be divided into 3 to 4 daily aliquots for subcutaneous fluid administration provided the patient is not severely dehydrated or volume limits are not exceeded.

Fluid Types

In choosing the most appropriate fluid for IV use, one should consider the acid-base status of the patient, the tonicity of the patient's serum, and the patient's serum electrolyte concentrations. Normal plasma osmolality in dogs and cats ranges from 290 to 330 mOsm/L. Diseases that alter sodium or glucose concentrations also affect a patient's plasma osmolality. The patient's parameters are assessed in reference to the pH, osmolality, and electrolyte composition of the available crystalloid fluid types. There is no perfect fluid choice for a specific patient, but a working knowledge of patient parameters, fluid solution characteristics, and clinical experience guide fluid selection.

Hypotonic fluids diffuse out of the vasculature faster than isotonic or hypertonic solutions following administration, and overzealous administration can cause red blood cells (RBCs) to swell and lyse. Administration of hypertonic solutions can cause phlebitis and RBC crenation, possibly affecting RBC functions. Replacement fluids (**Figure**) should be used to treat shock (electrolyte concentration similar to plasma) and to correct dehydration. Maintenance fluids are designed to replace normal daily losses of electrolytes (40–60 mEq of sodium/L, 15–20mEq of potassium/L) and should be used once electrolyte imbalances and dehydration have been corrected.

Replacement Fluids — Selected Topics

Many different types of replacement fluids are commercially available. In most situations their use is interchangeable. However, there are clinical situations where the use of a specific replacement fluid is the treatment of choice.

Normal Saline (0.9% sodium chloride) Solution

Normal (0.9%) saline solution has a pH of 5.5 and 154 mEq of sodium and chloride/L, and has a higher osmolality than most other replacement fluid types, due to the higher sodium concentration. Normal saline solution is the fluid of choice for hypercalcemic patients. Administration of sodium chloride promotes calciuresis as the sodium ion competes with the calcium ion for reabsorption in the renal tubules, resulting in less calcium ion being reabsorbed. Additionally, animals with metabolic alkalosis should be treated with normal saline solution (see Chapter 17). Saline administration is often recommended for short-term stabilization of patients with life-threatening hyperkalemia, such as addisonian crisis or urinary tract obstruction. However, these patients are often markedly acidotic, and prolonged administration of normal saline might perpetuate the acidosis and electrolyte disorders. Acidosis tends to promote translocation of potassium from the intracellular to the intravascular spaces in exchange for hydrogen ion. Because saline is an acidifying solution, extended therapy in patients with non-life-threatening or resolving hyperkalemia should involve administration of LRS, Plasma-lyte A, or Normosol R. Finally normal saline solution is the fluid of choice for most CRIs as it has few drug interactions.

LRS

LRS has a pH of 6.5, lower sodium and chloride concentrations, and higher calcium, potassium, and lactate concentrations, compared to normal saline solution. Owing to its pH, LRS is a good choice for a replacement fluid. Most animals with dehydration or in hypovolemic shock have a mild to moderate metabolic acidosis, due to hypoperfusion of tissues and the accumulation of lactic acid. Since the pH of 0.9% saline is 5.5, its administration can worsen acidosis initially. Profound acidosis often accompanies metabolic conditions such as DKA and the use of LRS for replacement fluid therapy is indicated. However, there are a few clinical situations where the use of LRS is contraindicated. The calcium contained in LRS may activate the coagulation cascade. Therefore, LRS should never be administered through the same delivery set as a blood transfusion. Similarly, given its calcium content, LRS should not be used to treat hypercalcemia. LRS or any lactate-containing fluid should also be used judiciously in patients with liver failure, because of an impaired ability to convert lactate to bicarbonate. Similarly, the IV administration of any lactate-containing IV fluids in dogs with lymphoma may elevate the already supernormal lactate levels in these patients.

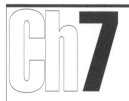

Disorders of Calcium I: Calcium Metabolism and Hypercalcemia

Lilian Cornejo and Alison R. Gaynor

A

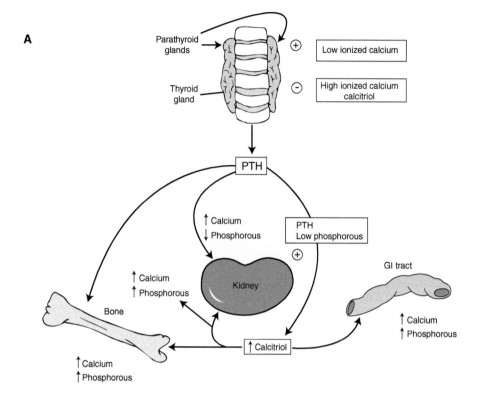

Parathyroid glands

Thyroid gland

(+) Low ionized calcium

(−) High ionized calcium calcitriol

PTH

↑ Calcium
↓ Phosphorous

PTH
Low phosphorous
(+)

Kidney

↑ Calcium
↑ Phosphorous

Bone

↑ Calcium
↑ Phosphorous

GI tract

↑ Calcium
↑ Phosphorous

↑ Calcitriol

B Causes of Hypercalcemia

Neoplasia
  Lymphosarcoma
  Multiple myeloma
  Anal sac apocrine gland adenocarcinoma
  Mammary gland adenocarcinoma
  Prostatic adenocarcinoma
  Squamous cell carcinoma
  Bone neoplasia
          Primary
          Metastatic
Primary hyperparathyroidism
Hypoadrenocorticism
Hypervitaminosis
  Cholecalciferol rodenticide toxicosis
  Oversupplementation
  Plants [Cestrum diurnum
    (day-blooming jessamine), *Solanum* spp.]
  Calcipotreine ingestion (psoriasis
    medication)
Acute renal failure
Chronic renal failure
Skeletal disorders
  Osteomyelitis (bacterial, fungal)
  Hypertrophic osteodystrophy
  Disuse osteoporosis
Physiologic
  Young growing animals
Spurious
  Hemolysis
  Lipemia
  Postprandial
  Laboratory error

C Clinical Manifestations of Hypercalcemia

Renal
  Isothenuria
  Polyuria/polydipsia
  Azotemia
          Prerenal
          Renal
  Decreased renal blood flow
  Nephrocalcinosis
  Interstitial nephritis
Neuromuscular
  Depression
  Lethargy
  Seizures
  Coma
  Muscle weakness
  Depressed deep tendon reflexes
Cardiovascular
  Prolonged PR interval
  Shortened QT interval
  Cardiac arrhythmias
  Increased cardiac sensitivity to digitalis
  Hypertension
GI
  Anorexia
  Vomiting
  Gastroduodenal ulceration
  Pancreatitis

D Treatment of Hypercalcemia[a]

Volume Expansion/Calciuresis

0.9% NaCl[b]	100-125 mL/kg/day, IV
Furosemide	2-4 mg/kg q8-12h, PO, SQ, IV
	0.1-1.0 mg/kg/hr IV CRI

Inhibit Bone Resorption

Prednisone	1.0-2.2 mg/kg q12h, PO, SQ, IV
Dexamethasone	0.1-0.22 mg/kg q12h, SQ, IV (corticosteroids also inhibit intestinal calcium absorption, increase renal calcium excretion)
Calcitonin	4-6 IU/kg q8-12h, SQ

Other Miscellaneous Therapies

Biphosphonates (etidronate, pamidronate)- inhibit bone resorptiom
Plicamycin (Mithracin)- antineoplastic agent, inhibits bone resorption, many side effects
Cisplatin, gallium nitrate- antineoplastic agents, inhibit bone resorption, nephrotoxic
Prostaglandin synthesis inhibitors
Sodium bicarbonate
Calcium channel antagonists
Peritoneal dialysis/ Hemodialysis
Calcium-restricted diet

[a] See text for details
[b] Rough guide only. Actual rate will depend on patient's hydration status, degree of hypercalcemia, and degree of other organ impairment

The divalent cation calcium is an important homeostatic ion and is an integral component of teeth and bones. As a regulatory ion, calcium is vital for processes such as muscle contraction, neural excitation, blood coagulation, enzyme activity, hormonal secretion, and cell adhesion. Calcium is also an important regulator of cardiac excitation-contraction coupling and of vascular smooth-muscle tone, and plays critical roles in cellular second messenger systems and signal transduction.

Physiology

Ninety-nine percent of total body calcium is in bone, with the remainder distributed between intracellular and extracellular sites. Extracellular calcium exists in 3 forms: a physiologically active ionized form (50%); a protein-bound form (40%); and a chelated form complexed with bicarbonate, citrate, and lactate (10%). Distribution between these forms varies with pH, protein levels (particularly albumin), and amounts of chelators. Acidosis causes a shift in total calcium from protein-bound forms to the ionized form; with alkalosis, the opposite occurs.

Calcium homeostasis is regulated by intestinal absorption, renal excretion, and skeletal turnover, which in turn are influenced primarily by the actions of parathyroid hormone (PTH) and the active form of vitamin D_3 (1,25-dihydrocholecalciferol or calcitriol) (**Part A**). Normally 98% of the filtered calcium load is reabsorbed; most reabsorption occurs in the proximal convoluted tubule and thick ascending limb of the loop of Henle. The remainder is reabsorbed in the distal convoluted tubule under active regulation by PTH. PTH also stimulates skeletal calcium mobilization as well as calcitriol synthesis. Intestinal calcium absorption is regulated mainly by calcitriol, which also stimulates distal tubular calcium reabsorption and skeletal calcium mobilization and provides feedback to inhibit both its own production and that of PTH.

Diagnosis

Diagnosis of causes of calcium disorders depends on the patient's history, findings at physical examination, and results of screening laboratory tests, as well as ancillary tests such as PTH and PTH-rp measurements, lymph node biopsies, and bone marrow examination.

Total serum calcium concentration is measured routinely in veterinary laboratories, and determination of ionized calcium is becoming more available. Changes in total calcium often parallel changes in ionized calcium; however, particularly in critically ill patients, total calcium concentration may not be representative of true calcium status. In addition, hypoalbuminemia will decrease total calcium levels without necessarily affecting ionized calcium levels.

Pathophysiology

In general, causes of hypercalcemia usually result in a combination of increased bone resorption, increased intestinal absorption, and decreased renal calcium excretion (**Part B**). Malignant neoplasia is the most common cause of pathologic hypercalcemia. This paraneoplastic syndrome may be caused by circulating humoral and/or locally produced factors induced or secreted by tumor cells [PTH-related peptide (PTH-rp), PTH, calcitriol, prostaglandins, osteoclast activating factors, transforming growth factors, interleukins-1, -4, and -6, tumor necrosis factor (TNF)-α, TNF-β] that mainly cause increased osteoclastic bone resorption. Excessive and inappropriate PTH secretion by parathyroid adenomas or adenocarcinomas causes primary hyperparathyroidism. Acidosis, decreased GFR and increased renal tubular calcium reabsorption, and hypocortisolemia contribute to hypercalcemia associated with hypoadrenocorticism, although ionized calcium may be normal. Hypervitaminosis D can cause severe hypercalcemia, and often concurrent hyperphosphatemia, within 24 hours of ingestion. The mild hypercalcemia sometimes seen with renal failure may be caused by a number of factors, including decreased GFR, decreased renal PTH degradation, and an altered set-point for calcium suppression of PTH secretion.

Clinical Presentation

The presentation of animals with hypercalcemia ranges from asymptomatic to comatose with renal failure, depending on the degree, rate of development, and duration of hypercalcemia, in addition to underlying causes and other concurrent metabolic derangements (**Part C**). Polyuria and isosthenuria occur early, in part due to interference with the action of ADH on collecting duct cells. Polydipsia occurs secondary to polyuria, and by direct stimulation of the hypothalamic thirst center by hypercalcemia. In addition to causing renal vasoconstriction, which can result in ischemic tubular injury, hypercalcemia may result in renal mineralization and irreversible renal damage. Neuromuscular signs are thought to be secondary to depressed neuromuscular transmission, caused by increased intracellular calcium concentrations. Cardiovascular manifestations are due to direct positive inotropic and negative chronotropic effects of calcium, as well as cardiac mineralization and elevated catecholamine levels. Hypercalcemia can cause increased gastric acid secretion, contributing to gastroduodenal ulcer formation, and decreased GI motility. Patients with primary hyperparathyroidism tend to be middle aged and older, whereas those with hypercalcemia of malignancy and vitamin D toxicosis are more likely to present in a hypercalcemic crisis.

Treatment

Therapy for hypercalcemia is directed toward the underlying cause, correction of hypercalcemia, and supportive care for associated organ dysfunction. Clinical signs and the degree of hypercalcemia dictate how aggressively patients should be treated (**Part D**). Volume expansion with saline is a critical component of therapy. This will lower calcium levels by dilution in extracellular fluid, by correcting acidosis, and by causing calciuresis. Further diuresis with furosemide after volume expansion enhances calciuresis by interfering with calcium reabsorption in the loop of Henle. Urine output and levels of other electrolytes should be monitored carefully, and central venous pressure monitoring may be needed in patients with renal or cardiac insufficiency. Corticosteroids inhibit bone resorption and intestinal calcium absorption and are particularly effective in patients with vitamin D toxicoses. Dietary calcium restriction is also helpful in these conditions because of the long half-lives of vitamin D metabolites. Because corticosteroids are cytotoxic to malignant lymphocytes and can mask a diagnosis of lymphoma, they should not be used in cases in which a diagnosis has not been established. Calcitonin is also quite effective in rapidly lowering calcium levels in hypercalcemia in which bone resorption plays a large role. Calcium channel blockers may antagonize life-threatening cardiovascular signs until more definitive therapy can be pursued. Other therapeutic measures that may be indicated include biphosphonate administration, gastric decontamination in cases of intoxication, and peritoneal or hemodialysis in patients with oliguria.

Continued investigations into safe and efficacious agents for treatment of hypercalcemia may allow these products to be used in veterinary patients in the future.

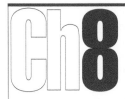

Disorders of Calcium II: Hypocalcemia

Lilian Cornejo and Alison R. Gaynor

A Causes of Hypocalcemia

Primary hypoparathyroidism
  Idiopathic/immune mediated
  Congenital atrophy

Secondary hypoparathyroidism

  Postparathyroidectomy
  Post thyroidectomy
  Cervical trauma

Hypomagnesemia

Redistribution
  Feline tetany (eclampsia)
  Massive trauma/rhabdomyolysis
  Phosphate enemas
  Rapid phosphorus infusion
  Sodium bicarbonate therapy
  Massive blood transfusion
  Ethylene glycol intoxication
  Acute pancreatitis
  Extensive IV fluid therapy

Renal failure

  Acute
  Chronic (renal secondary hyperparathyroidism)

Nutritional secondary hyperparathyroidism
Furosemide diuresis
Hypovitaminosis D
  Hepatic insufficiency
  Severe malabsorption/maldigestion

Sepsis/SIRS

B Clinical Manifestations of Hypocalcemia

Neuromuscular
  Muscle tremors/ fasciculations
  Hyperexcitability
  Restlessness
  Tetany
  Seizures
  Hyperthermia
  Panting
  Facial rubbing

Cardiovascular
  Prolonged QT interval

GI
  Anorexia
  Vomiting
  Diarrhea

C Treatment of Hypocalcemia[a]

Parenteral Calcium[b]
  Initial[c]:

10% calcium gluconate	0.5-1.5 mL/kg slow IV bolus over 10-30 min	
10% calcium chloride[d]	1.5-3.0 mL (total dose) slow IV bolus over 10-30 min	

  Subsequent:

10% calcium gluconate	0.5-1.5 mL/kg diluted with equal volume of saline. SQ, q6-8h	
	5-15 mg/kg/hr IV CRI	

Oral Vitamin D Preparations

Product	Dose	Peak Effect	Time for Toxicosis to Resolve
Calcitriol	0.02-0.03 mcg/kg/day	1-4 days	2-14 days
Dihydrotachysterol			
Initial	0.02-0.03 mg/kg/day	2-7 days	1-3 weeks
Maintenance	0.01-0.02 mg/kg q24-48h		
Ergocalciferol (vitamin D2)			
Initial	4000-6000 U/kg/day	5-21 days	1-18 weeks
Maintenance	1000-2000 U/kg qdq week		

Oral Calcium
  50-100 mg elemental calcium/kg/day divided q6-8h
    Many available formulations (calcium carbonate, calcium chloride, calcium gluconate, calcium lactate)

[a] See text for details
[b] Do not dilute in solutions containing bicarbonate, lactate or magnesium.
[c] Temporarily discontinue infusion if bradycardia or other arrhythmias noted.
[d] Extremely caustic if given perivascularly.

Pathophysiology

In general, hypocalcemia occurs with impaired secretion or action of PTH, impaired calcitriol synthesis or action, and changes in distribution (**Part A**). After parathyroidectomy for hyperparathyroidism, after bilateral thyroidectomy, and potentially after treatment for hypercalcemia of any cause, remaining parathyroid tissue may be atrophied and hypofunctional, thereby leading to hypocalcemia of variable duration. With eclampsia, increased demands for calcium during lactation in excess of that obtained from diet and from bone can cause acute hypocalcemia. Calcium supplementation during gestation exacerbates this tendency by suppressing PTH before the acute calcium demands of lactation occur. Acute hyperphosphatemia in feline urinary tract obstruction, acute renal failure, and other disorders causes hypocalcemia by the law of mass action. With chronic renal failure (CRF), hypocalcemia may occur secondary to hyperphosphatemia, decreased calcitriol production, and increased renal calcium loss. Alkalinization with sodium bicarbonate causes a shift from ionized to protein-bound calcium, and also direct chelation of calcium with bicarbonate, and can precipitate a hypocalcemic crisis in patients with mild or subclinical hypocalcemia. Chelation of calcium to citrate after multiple blood transfusions may cause clinical hypocalcemia, particularly in patients with defective citrate metabolism (hepatic or renal insufficiency, hypothermia). Chelation of calcium to the metabolite oxalate with subsequent calcium oxalate precipitation can cause severe hypocalcemia in ethylene glycol toxicosis. Extensive IV fluid therapy and furosemide may exacerbate hypocalcemic tendencies by dilution (IV fluids) and by natriuresis, which induces calciuresis. Ionized hypocalcemia associated with sepsis and the systemic inflammatory response syndrome (SIRS) is common in critically ill humans, although it has not been reported in veterinary patients. Multifactorial causes include acquired abnormalities in PTH and Vitamin D synthesis and action, acquired and preexisting changes in renal and GI function, electrolyte derangements such as hypomagnesemia, elevated levels of pro-inflammatory cytokines, extensive fluid and diuretic therapy, blood transfusions, and inadequate nutritional support.

Clinical Presentation

The clinical presentation of hypocalcemic patients depends on the degree of hypocalcemia and the rate of its development, in addition to the underlying cause. Since hypocalcemia increases membrane excitability by enhancing sodium influx, most clinical signs of acute hypocalcemia are associated with increased neuromuscular activity (**Part B**). Clinicians should keep in mind, however, that these signs can be masked by other concurrent electrolyte derangements such as hyperkalemia or hypokalemia, and by acidosis. Correction of acidosis in a patient with marginal hypocalcemia can precipitate a hypocalcemic crisis. Patients with severe or prolonged tetany or seizure activity may become dangerously hyperthermic, and may present with severe metabolic and neurologic derangements. With secondary hypoparathyroidism, clinical hypocalcemia may develop 1–5 days postoperatively. Eclampsia typically occurs in small-breed dogs, 1–4 weeks post partum.

Treatment

Patients exhibiting clinical signs of hypocalcemia should receive parenteral calcium (**Part C**) as well as supportive therapy. Either calcium gluconate or calcium chloride can be given as a slow IV bolus over 10–30 minutes with concurrent ECG monitoring. Overdosing or too rapid administration can lead to cardiac arrest. Additional infusions may be necessary in some patients; alternatively, calcium gluconate may be administered subcutaneously or as a constant-rate IV infusion. Ionized calcium concentrations should be monitored carefully. Calcium levels should be corrected to just below normal, to avoid calciuresis and to maintain a stimulus for PTH secretion. Dogs with eclampsia should have their puppies weaned immediately and should receive a balanced diet. Patients with primary hypoparathyroidism and others at risk for continued hypocalcemia should receive oral vitamin D supplementation. Because of variability in vitamin D preparations and in individual patient responses to therapy, calcium levels should be monitored periodically. Oral calcium supplementation, although often unnecessary, may also be used. Calcium in any form should not be administered to hyperphosphatemic patients until after correction of the hyperphosphatemia.

The Future

With the development and availability of point-of-care testing, measurement of ionized calcium levels should become routine in veterinary medicine. Techniques for measurement of protein-bound and chelated forms of calcium are available experimentally and may allow better understanding of the shifts between forms of calcium in various disease states, particularly in critically ill cats and dogs.

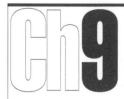

Disorders of Phosphorus I: Phosphorus Metabolism and Hyperphosphatemia

Alison R. Gaynor and Lilian Cornejo

A

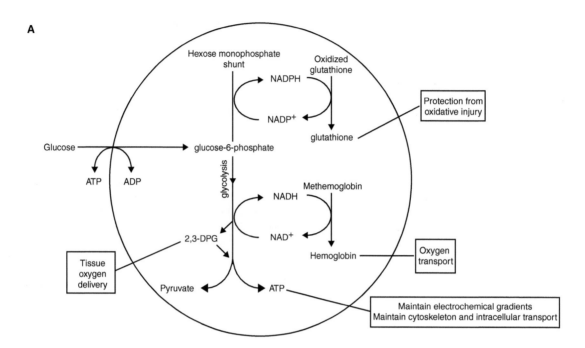

B Causes of Hyperphosphatemia

Redistribution
    Massive cellular damage
        Massive tissue trauma/rhabdomyolysis
        Severe hemolysis
        Tumor lysis syndrome
        Thromboembolism
        Snakebite
    Metabolic acidosis

Decreased renal excretion
    Azotemia
        Prerenal
        Postrenal (urinary tract obstruction or rupture)
        Renal
         ARF
         CRF

    Endocrine
        Hypoparathyroidism
        Hypersomatotropism
        Hyperthyroidism

Increased intake
    GI
        Phosphate-containing enemas
        Phosphate-containing urinary acidifiers
        Hypervitaminosis D
         Cholecalciferol rodenticide toxicosis
         Oversupplementation
         Plants [*Cestrum diurnum* (day-blooming jessamine), *Solanum* spp]
         Calcipiotriene ingestion (psoriasis medication)
        Ethylene glycol toxicosis (phosphate containing rust inhibitors)
    Physiologic
        Young, growing animals

Laboratory error
        Hemolysis
        Hyperlipidemia
        Hyperproteinemia

Phosphorus has an integral role in the structure and function of all cells. As a component of adenosine triphosphate (ATP), phosphorus is critical in energy production and in helping to supply the energy needed for essential processes such as nerve conduction, muscle contraction, and epithelial transport. Phosphorus is a component of phospholipids and of 2,3-diphosphoglycerate (2,3-DPG) and thus plays an important role in the maintenance of cell membrane integrity as well as peripheral oxygen delivery. It is also important in nucleic acid, protein, fat, and carbohydrate metabolism; in cellular second messenger systems and signal transduction; and as a urinary buffer (**Part A**).

Physiology

Phosphate is the major intracellular anion. Eighty-five percent to 90% of total body phosphorus is present in bone as hydroxyapatite, with most of the remaining 10%–15% in soft tissues. Serum phosphorus constitutes <1% of total-body phosphorus and is composed of protein-bound forms (10%–20%), free anionic forms, and forms complexed to sodium, magnesium, or calcium.

Serum phosphorus concentration is regulated by dietary intake, renal excretion, interactions of the hormones vitamin D and PTH, and factors that promote cellular translocation such as pH, glucose, and insulin. Intestinal phosphate absorption occurs primarily in the jejunum and is enhanced by the active form of vitamin D (1,25-dihydrocholecalciferol or calcitriol). Low dietary phosphate levels result in increased renal production of calcitriol, leading to increased intestinal and renal phosphate absorption. Renal phosphate excretion is regulated by GFR and the maximum tubular transport rate (T_mP) for phosphate (normally 80%–90% of the filtered phosphate load is reabsorbed). Reabsorption is sodium dependent, occurs primarily in the proximal convoluted tubule, and is decreased by PTH, which decreases T_mP.

Diagnosis

Serum phosphate is measured as inorganic phosphate and is reported as elemental phosphorus (in mg/dL) (3.1 mg of phosphorus/dL = 1.0 mmol of phosphorus/L = 1.8 mEq of phosphate/L). Although serum phosphorus concentration does not reliably reflect total-body phosphorus status, it does appear to correlate well with the clinical manifestations of hypophosphatemia and hyperphosphatemia. Clinicians should maintain a high index of suspicion for hypophosphatemia in patients and situations that predispose to its development (see next chapter). For example, because of metabolic acidosis, osmotic effects of hyperglycemia, and renal insufficiency, serum phosphorus concentrations in animals with DKA may be normal or even elevated, despite total-body phosphorus depletion.

Pathophysiology

Increased phosphorus intake, decreased renal excretion, and redistribution of phosphate from intracellular to extracellular sites may result in hyperphosphatemia (**Part B**). Renal failure, particularly acute renal failure (ARF), where compensatory mechanisms have not had time to develop, is one of the more common causes of hyperphosphatemia in veterinary medicine. In chronic renal failure (CRF), significant hyperphosphatemia occurs when the GFR has decreased to <20% of normal (prior to that, tubular compensatory mechanisms ameliorate the tendency toward elevations in phosphorus that occur due to a declining GFR). Metabolic acidosis causes extracellular phosphate translocation. Release of intracellular phosphorus to the extracellular space occurs with massive cellular damage such as that seen with major trauma or thromboembolic disease (both before and after thrombolytic therapy). Additionally, myoglobinuria-induced ARF may exacerbate hyperphosphatemia in this situation. Growth hormone and thyroxine increase renal tubular phosphate reabsorption. Iatrogenic sources and various toxicoses are also significant causes of hyperphosphatemia in veterinary critical care medicine.

Clinical Presentation

With hyperphosphatemia, the clinical presentation depends on the underlying cause and the rate of development of hyperphosphatemia. Because the calcium phosphate solubility product ($[Ca] \times [P]$) must remain constant, increases in serum phosphorus concentration lead to reciprocal decreases in serum ionized calcium concentration. Therefore, many of the clinical signs of hyperphosphatemia, particularly that developing acutely, are related to hypocalcemia and include tetany and soft-tissue mineralization (when $[Ca] \times [P] \geq 60$). Hypotension and diarrhea may also be noted (see Chapter 4). Hyperphosphatemia stimulates renal secondary hyperparathyroidism, thus contributing to the progression of CRF. Animals with advanced CRF may exhibit fibrous osteodystrophy from increased PTH-stimulated osteoclastic bone resorption, as well as other signs secondary to uremia.

Treatment

Treatment for hyperphosphatemia should be directed toward correcting the underlying cause. Exogenous sources of phosphate and vitamin D should be discontinued. Phosphate-containing enemas are contraindicated in cats and small dogs and should be used with extreme caution, if at all, in larger dogs. Clinicians must anticipate (and attempt to avoid) situations that may predispose to hyperphosphatemia. For example, IV fluid diuresis prior to and during initiation of chemotherapy in animals with lymphosarcoma suspected to have large tumor burdens may be beneficial. IV fluid therapy with 0.9% sodium chloride is the mainstay of treatment for animals with hyperphosphatemia. In addition to diluting phosphate in the extracellular fluid, volume expansion will help correct acidosis and will increase renal phosphate excretion secondary to an increased GFR and to natriuresis. In emergent situations, addition of dextrose (1.0 gm/kg, IV) and if necessary, insulin (0.5 U/kg, IV) will temporarily decrease serum phosphorus concentration. Animals with chronic hyperphosphatemia should receive phosphate-restricted diets (achieved mainly by protein restriction), as well as oral phosphate binders to decrease intestinal phosphate absorption. Magnesium-containing products should be avoided in animals with renal insufficiency.

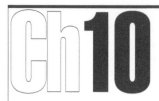

Disorders of Phosphorus II: Hypophosphatemia

Alison R. Gaynor and Lilian Cornejo

A Causes of Hypophosphatemia

Redistribution
  Carbohydrate load and/or insulin administration
  Nutritional recovery syndrome
  Insulin therapy in DKA
  Respiratory alkalosis (hyperventilation)
  Hypothermia
  Sepsis
Decreased renal reabsorption
  Primary hyperparathyroidism
  Renal tubular disorders (Fanconi's syndrome, others)
  Proximal tubular diuretics
  Hyperadrenocorticism
  Eclampsia
  Diuresis
          IV fluid administration
          Osmotic diuresis (glucose, mannitol)
Decreased intestinal absorption
  Dietary deficiency
  Vomiting
  Malabsorption syndromes
  Phosphate binders/antacids (e.g. aluminum hydroxide, sucralfate)
  Hypovitaminosis D
Laboratory error
  Mannitol

B Systemic Effects of Hypophosphatemia

Hematologic
  Erythrocytes
          Increased fragility
          Hemolysis
          Impaired tissue oxygen delivery
  Leukocytes
          Impaired chemotaxis, phagocytosis, and bacterial activity
  Platelets
          Decreased survival
          Decreased clot retraction
          Thrombocytopenia

Muscular
  Generalized muscle weakness
  Myalgia
  Rhabdomyolysis
  Decreased cardiac contractility

Neurologic
  Metabolic encephalopathy
  Paresthesias
  Ataxia
  Seizures
  Coma

GI
  Intestinal ileus
  Anorexia
  Nausea
  Vomiting

Skeletal
  Bone demineralization (chronic hypophosphatemia)

C Treatment of Hypophosphatemia[a]

IV replacement
  Potassium phosphate [b]: 3.0 mmol phosphate/mL
  and 4.3 mEq potassium/mL

        0.01–0.03 mmol/kg/hr for 6 hr,[c,d]

        0.06–0.10 mmol/kg/hr for 6–24hr [e]

Monitor serum phosphorus concentration q6h.
Discontinue when serum phosphorus concentration is ≥ 2.0–2.5 mg/dL

Oral replacement: 0.5–2.0 mmol/kg/24 hr
  Dairy products (milk : 0.029 mmol phosphorus/mL)
  Calcium phosphate tablets (580 mg calcium,
  450 mg phosphorus, 400 IU vitamin D3)
  Many other oral supplements

[a] see text for details
[b] very hypertonic-must be diluted in non-calcium-containing fluids.
[c] All doses given as a continous-rate IV infusion.
[d] Traditional dose recommendation.
[e] May be necessary for animals with severe phosphorus depletion.

Pathophysiology

Hypophosphatemia can result from the shifting of phosphate from extracellular to intracellular sites, from decreased intestinal or renal phosphate absorption, or from combinations of these factors (**Part A**).

Administration of a carbohydrate load (e.g., 5% dextrose) stimulates insulin secretion, which facilitates the transport of glucose and phosphate into cells where glucose is rapidly phosphorylated to glycolytic intermediates. Respiratory alkalosis (hyperventilation) stimulates glycolysis by activating phosphofructokinase. Nutritional support (enteral or parenteral routes, also sometimes dextrose infusions) in a malnourished animal with depleted total-body phosphorus stimulates accelerated rates of tissue repair as phosphorus is rapidly incorporated into cells or is used for energy production. Animals with DKA have total-body phosphorus deficits secondary to anorexia, decreased muscle mass, chronic hypoinsulinemia (impaired tissue utilization of phosphate), and urinary phosphate losses. Therapeutic interventions with insulin and IV fluids exacerbate or unmask hypophosphatemia and may precipitate a hypophosphatemic crisis. Diuretics acting at the proximal tubule may cause increased urinary excretion of phosphate secondary to natriuresis. Hypovitaminosis D causes decreased intestinal phosphate absorption, as well as increased renal losses secondary to the increased levels of PTH stimulated by hypocalcemia. Hypophosphatemia also may be an early sign of sepsis, possibly related to the hypermetabolic state or respiratory alkalosis.

Clinical Presentation

The clinical presentation of hypophosphatemic animals depends on the underlying disease process, as well as the degree of hypophosphatemia and the rate of its development. Because of the high energy requirements of erythrocytes, skeletal muscle cells, and cerebral cells, most clinical signs of acute hypophosphatemia are related to cellular ATP depletion in these body systems (**Part B**). Loss of membrane deformability in erythrocytes results in reticuloendothelial clearance of these more rigid cells, which are also prone to osmotic lysis secondary to impaired Na^+, K^+-ATPase pump function. Hypophosphatemic animals may be more susceptible to infections and may exhibit bleeding tendencies. Animals with acute, severe hypophosphatemia may demonstrate acute hemolytic anemia, muscle weakness (including muscles involved with ventilation) and rhabdomyolysis,

and seizures, obtundation, and coma. Clinically significant hypophosphatemia is most commonly seen after initiation of insulin therapy in animals with DKA and with refeeding of chronically malnourished animals (e.g., cats with hepatic lipidosis). Clinical signs, particularly hemolysis, seem to develop with relatively milder degrees of hypophosphatemia in cats as compared to dogs.

Treatment

One of the most important aspects of therapy for hypophosphatemia is anticipation (and avoidance or correction, if possible) of predisposing situations, as previously discussed. Feeding of malnourished animals should be increased gradually to the full caloric requirement over several days, and high-carbohydrate diets should be avoided. Animals receiving phosphate binders should be monitored carefully. Sucralfate should not be administered to animals with proven or suspected phosphate deficits. Phosphorus-deficient patients requiring transfusions should receive only fresh whole blood or packed RBCs, because the diminished levels of 2,3-DPG in stored blood products may precipitate a hypophosphatemic crisis.

IV phosphate supplementation is recommended for patients demonstrating clinical signs or for those whose serum phosphorus is ≤1.5 mg/dL (**Part C**). Animals with severe depletion (DKA, nutritional recovery syndrome) may require higher doses and longer duration of treatment than the traditionally recommended dose. Potential complications of IV therapy include acute hypocalcemia, tetany, hyperphosphatemia, soft-tissue mineralization, and hypotension secondary to rapid infusion. Oral phosphate supplementation is safer and is recommended for animals with mild to moderate degrees of hypophosphatemia that are not exhibiting clinical signs. Phosphate administration in any form is contraindicated in oliguric or hypercalcemic patients.

The Future

Clinically significant alterations of phosphorus are becoming more frequently recognized in veterinary medicine. Hypophosphatemia, previously considered uncommon, is now associated with significant morbidity and mortality in critically ill cats and dogs. Continued investigations into the relationship of hypophosphatemia and sepsis, as well as the role phosphorus may play in other disorders, may provide better understanding of disease mechanisms and will enhance our ability to diagnose and treat these disorders.

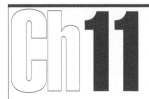

Disorders of Magnesium I: Magnesium Metabolism and Hypermagnesemia

Alison R. Gaynor and Lilian Cornejo

A Causes of Hypermagnesemia

Decreased glomerular filtration
  ARF
  CRF
  Prerenal azotemia

Endocrinopathies
  Hypoadrenocorticism
  Hyperparathyroidism
  Hypothyroidism

Iatrogenic overdose
  Antacids
  Cathartics
  Laxatives

B Treatment of Hypermagnesemia

Agent	Dose	Route
0.9% NaCl	100-125 mL/kg/day	IV
Furosemide	2-4 mg/kg q8-12h	PO, SQ, IV
	or	
	0.1-1.0 mg/kg/hr as CRI	IV
Calcium gluconate	5-15 mg/kg	IV (slowly)
	followed by 5-15 mg/kg/hr as CRI	IV (if necessary)
Physostigmine	0.02 mg/kg q12h	IV

Magnesium is the second most abundant intracellular cation. An essential dietary element, magnesium is a catalyst for >300 enzymes and is required for all cellular and metabolic functions involved in the generation and use of ATP. Magnesium is a cofactor for the membrane-bound Na^+/K^+-ATPase, Ca^{2+}-ATPase, and proton pumps and is thus necessary for maintenance of transmembrane potential and cell membrane function and integrity. In addition to transfer, storage, and utilization of energy, magnesium plays key roles in muscle contraction; regulation of vascular smooth muscle tone; nucleic acid synthesis; protein, fat, and carbohydrate metabolism; and cellular second messenger systems and signal transduction. Magnesium also may play a role in lymphocyte activation and cytokine production. Disorders of magnesium are becoming more frequently recognized in both human and veterinary medicine, and in fact may be among the most prevalent electrolyte abnormalities in critically ill animals.

Physiology

Sixty percent of total-body magnesium is in bone; 20%, within skeletal muscle; and the remainder, within the heart, liver, and other tissues. One-third of the skeletal magnesium compartment serves as an exchangeable reservoir for maintenance of a normal extracellular magnesium concentration. Serum magnesium constitutes only about 1% of total-body magnesium and is composed of a physiologically active ionized fraction (70%), a protein-bound fraction (20%), and a chelated fraction complexed with citrate, phosphate, and other anions (10%).

Magnesium homeostasis is regulated primarily by intestinal absorption and renal excretion. No primary regulatory hormone has been identified for magnesium homeostasis, although the adrenal, thyroid, and parathyroid glands may be involved. Intestinal absorption occurs primarily in the jejunum and ileum and is inversely proportional to the amount of magnesium ingested. Absorption is enhanced by active vitamin D and is impaired in the presence of diets containing large amounts of free fatty acids, phosphate, oxalate, and fiber; in addition, dietary calcium and magnesium may interfere with each other's absorption.

Regulation of serum magnesium and of total-body magnesium content is achieved mainly by the kidneys via glomerular filtration and tubular reabsorption. Thirty percent of filtered magnesium is passively reabsorbed in the proximal convoluted tubule, and 60%–65% is actively reabsorbed in the thick ascending limb of the loop of Henle. Regulation of renal magnesium handling is thought to occur primarily at the latter site, although the exact mechanism is undefined. Renal magnesium reabsorption is decreased in response to higher filtered loads and conversely, is increased in deficiency states.

Diagnosis

Determination of serum magnesium concentration is the most readily available technique for estimation of magnesium status. However, this may not accurately reflect total-body magnesium status, since serum magnesium represents <1% of total-body stores. Reported reference ranges for serum magnesium in dogs are 1.89–2.51 mg/dL and 1.7–2.4 mg/dL. Low serum magnesium levels are predictive of magnesium deficits; however, magnesium depletion also may exist despite normal serum levels. Alternatively, elevated serum magnesium levels do reflect increased body stores, although the exact correlation has not been determined. Physiologic tests for magnesium depletion such as 24-hour magnesium excretion and a parenteral magnesium tolerance test are available but may be impractical in an emergent setting. Measurement of ionized magnesium, the physiologically active fraction, may provide a more accurate reflection of intracellular ionized magnesium status, although veterinary clinical experience with this technique is limited at this time. The canine reference range for ionized magnesium is 1.07–1.46 mg/dL. Changes in serum magnesium seem to parallel changes in ionized magnesium. Clinicians should maintain a high index of suspicion for hypomagnesemia in critically ill patients with diseases (and/or therapeutic modalities) that predispose to magnesium depletion, particularly those with DKA or cardiovascular disease, as described in the next chapter. The presence of other concurrent electrolyte abnormalities, especially if refractory to replacement therapy, also should alert clinicians to the possibility of hypomagnesemia in these patients.

Pathophysiology

Since the normal kidney can easily eliminate large loads of magnesium, hypermagnesemia in the absence of azotemia is unusual. In fact, most clinical cases of hypermagnesemia involve varying degrees of renal insufficiency, particularly ARF (**Part A**). Animals with severe prerenal azotemia also may be hypermagnesemic. Certain endocrinopathies can cause a milder degree of hypermagnesemia through poorly understood mechanisms. Iatrogenic hypermagnesemia often involves improper dosing or failure to consider underlying renal function.

Clinical Presentation

The clinical presentation of hypermagnesemic patients depends on the degree of hypermagnesemia. Cardiovascular manifestations include prolongation of the PR interval and widening of the QRS complex at relatively lower levels of hypermagnesemia, because of delayed atrioventricular (AV) and interventricular conduction. Complete AV block and asystole may occur with severely elevated magnesium levels. Refractory hypotension secondary to relaxation of vascular resistance vessels has also been reported, as well as impaired blood clotting abilities.

Hypermagnesemia causes decreased impulse transmission across the neuromuscular junction, decreased postsynaptic membrane responsiveness, and an elevated threshold for axonal stimulation, all leading to various degrees of neuromuscular blockade. Loss of deep tendon reflexes is one of the earliest signs of magnesium toxicosis, and monitoring of these reflexes is recommended during acute therapy with parenteral magnesium. Extreme hypermagnesemia suppresses the release of acetylcholine at neuromuscular junctions and in the autonomic nervous system, causing respiratory muscle paralysis, vascular collapse, and death.

Treatment

The most important aspect of therapy for hypermagnesemia is discontinuation of any exogenous magnesium. Additional therapy depends on the degree of hypermagnesemia, clinical signs, and renal function (**Part B**). For patients with non-life-threatening hypermagnesemia and functional kidneys, the first line of therapy is diuresis with saline and loop diuretics. Hemodialysis or peritoneal dialysis may be required in patients with severely compromised renal function. With severe hypermagnesemia, intubation and mechanical ventilation may be necessary, as well as parenteral calcium to antagonize cardiotoxicity. In addition, anticholinesterases such as physostigmine may help ameliorate neuromuscular signs. Resuscitation efforts may be particularly difficult, since hypermagnesemic shock may be refractory to therapy with pressors such as epinephrine. Intense monitoring and correction of underlying causes of hypermagnesemia, if possible, are critical to outcome in patients with hypermagnesemia.

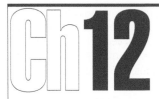

Disorders of Magnesium II: Hypomagnesemia

Alison R. Gaynor and Lilian Cornejo

A Causes of Hypomagnesemia

Gastrointestinal
  Reduced intake
        Prolonged starvation
        Prolonged IV fluid therapy
  Reduced absorption
        Diffuse small-intestinal disease
        Chronic diarrhea
        Extensive intestinal resection
        Pancreatic insufficiency
        Cholestatic liver disease

Renal
  Intrinsic tubular disorders
        ARF (polyuric phase)
        Renal tubular acidosis
        Postobstructive diuresis
  Drug-induced losses
        Loop diuretics, aminoglycosides, amphotericin B, digitalis, cisplatin, cyclosporine, ethanol
  Endocrinopathies
        Hyperthyroidism
        Hypoparathyroidism
  Other causes of tubular losses
        Osmotic diuresis (glucose, mannitol)
        Hypercalcemia
        Hypophosphatemia
        Extracellular fluid volume expansion
Redistribution
  Insulin administration
  Hyperadrenergic states (shock, sepsis, trauma, hypothermia)
  Acute pancreatitis
  Multiple blood transfusions
  Nutritional recovery syndrome
Other losses
  Severe burns
  Lactation
  Sweating

B Clinical Manifestations of Hypomagnesemia

Cardiovascular
  Ventricular arrhythmias: ventricular contractions, ventricular
    tachycardia, torsades de pointes, ventricular fibrillation
  Atrial arrhythmias (atrial tachycardia, atrial fibrillation)
  Digitalis-induced arrhythmias
  Hypertension
Metabolic
  Hypokalemia
  Hypocalcemia
  Hyponatremia
Neuromuscular
  Muscle weakness
        Generalized
        Focal
           Dyspnea
           Dysphagia
  Muscle fasciculations
  Hyperreflexia
  Ataxia
  Mental depression
  Seizures
  Coma
Hematologic
  Altered platelet aggregation
  Anemia
GI
  Anorexia
  Nausea
  Ileus

C Acute Treatment of Hypomagnesemia[a]

Acute management[b,c]

  0.75-1.00 mEq/kg/day for 1-2 days, then 0.3-0.5 mEq/kg/day for 2-5 days

Life-threatening Ventricular Arrhythmias

  0.15-0.30 mEq/kg over 5-15 min IV

Elemental Magnesium: 1 mM = 2 mEq = 24 mg

Parenteral Magnesium Formulations
  50% Magnesium sulfate: 8.13 mEq/ gm
  50% Magnesium chloride: 9.25 mEq/gm

[a] See text for details.
[b] All doses given as a continuous-rate IV infusion in 5% dextrose in water.
[c] Do not administer magnesium in fluids containing calcium, lactate, or bicarbonate.

Pathophysiology

Magnesium deficiency may result from decreased intake or absorption, increased losses (primarily renal), or changes in distribution (see **Part A**). A combination of these factors may lead to hypomagnesemia in conditions such as DKA, and may be exacerbated further by therapeutic intervention. Renal magnesium losses play a key role in the development of hypomagnesemia and occur by various direct and indirect mechanisms, including drug-induced enhancement of renal magnesium loss, a particularly important consideration in critically ill animals. Insulin administration results in shifts of magnesium from extracellular to intracellular sites in a manner similar to its effects on potassium and phosphate. Hyperadrenergic states also may cause intracellular shifting of magnesium, as well as chelation of magnesium by increased levels of circulating free fatty acids secondary to β-adrenergic stimulation of lipolysis. Magnesium also is chelated by citrated blood products administered in large quantities. Hypomagnesemia secondary to fat saponification has been associated with acute pancreatitis. Critically ill animals may be at increased risk for hypomagnesemia because of stress, catabolic disease, aggressive IV fluid therapy, nasogastric suctioning, peritoneal dialysis and hemodialysis, total parenteral nutrition, diuretics, and multiple blood transfusions.

Clinical Presentation

The clinical presentation of animals with hypomagnesemia is variable and may be a direct consequence of magnesium deficiency or secondary to other concurrent electrolyte abnormalities. Patients may have 1 or more signs (**Part B**) or may be completely asymptomatic. Cardiovascular manifestations include various atrial and ventricular arrhythmias, particularly torsades de pointes, a form of ventricular tachycardia. Magnesium deficiency may inhibit function of the Na^+/K^+-ATPase pump, leading to decreased intracellular potassium concentrations and a decreased ratio of intracellular to extracellular potassium, which in turn decreases the resting membrane potential and predisposes to arrhythmia generation. Additive effects on the Na^+K^+ pump also lead to enhanced sensitivity to toxic effects of cardiac glycosides and predispose patients to digitalis-induced arrhythmias. The potential for arrhythmia generation may be exacerbated further by renal magnesium and potassium losses secondary to the common use of loop diuretics in patients with cardiovascular disease. Dogs with cardiovascular disease are at increased risk for hypomagnesemia, although a causal relationship has not been identified.

Metabolic manifestations include hypokalemia or hypocalcemia, or both, that may be refractory to replacement therapy without concurrent correction of magnesium depletion. Hyponatremia also may be seen. Hypokalemia is the most common electrolyte abnormality associated with hypomagnesemia, occurring in as many as 73% of critically ill hypomagnesemic cats and dogs. Losses of both potassium and magnesium may be due to a common underlying disorder (DKA, diuretics); however, magnesium deficiency can lead to potassium depletion by causing an inappropriate kaliuresis secondary to decreased proximal tubular potassium reabsorption and enhanced distal tubular secretion. With concurrent hypokalemia, hypomagnesemia may manifest as focal or generalized muscle weakness. Magnesium deficiency alone causes increased neuromuscular excitability because of increased release of acetylcholine at axon terminals, as well as increased skeletal muscle calcium content. With concurrent hypocalcemia, hypomagnesemia may present as muscle fasciculations, ataxia, or seizure activity. Low magnesium concentrations may impair adenylate cyclase activity, leading to refractory hypocalcemia secondary to impaired secretion of PTH, decreased synthesis of PTH, and end-organ resistance to the actions of PTH.

Treatment

Mild nonclinical hypomagnesemia may resolve with treatment of the underlying disease process. Magnesium supplementation is recommended if serum magnesium is <1.2 mg/dL, and in patients with higher serum levels that are exhibiting clinical signs or that have concurrent electrolyte disorders. Supplementation should be avoided in patients with cardiac conduction abnormalities and should be decreased by 50%–75% of the calculated dose in the presence of azotemia. For acute management, magnesium is administered as an IV continuous-rate infusion (CRI) (**Part C**), followed by a lower dose for several days because complete magnesium repletion occurs slowly. Supplementation should be tailored to the needs of the individual patient. Magnesium levels and deep tendon reflexes should be monitored at least once a day during supplementation. Levels of other electrolytes, particularly potassium, also should be monitored carefully, and potassium supplementation may need to be decreased after several hours of magnesium replacement. For treatment of life-threatening ventricular arrhythmias and digitalis-induced arrhythmias, magnesium is administered as a slow IV bolus to raise the ventricular fibrillation threshold. Magnesium overdoses can cause hypocalcemia, hypotension, AV and bundle branch blocks, and respiratory muscle weakness (Chapter 7). Oral magnesium supplementation may be beneficial for chronic management of dogs on long-term digitalis and diuretics. The suggested dose is 1–2 mEq/kg/day of either magnesium hydroxide or magnesium oxide. The main side effect is diarrhea.

The Future

Currently, most veterinary knowledge about disorders of magnesium is based on information derived from human studies and from limited studies in critically ill animals. More routine determination of serum and ionized magnesium levels in sick cats and dogs may allow better characterization of these disorders. Development of techniques to better evaluate intracellular magnesium status, such as lymphocyte magnesium content, also may help increase our understanding of these disorders. Furthermore, this may lead to more accurate dosing regimens rather than the current practice of supplementing magnesium empirically. Finally, results of experimental investigations in canine models of shock, cardiopulmonary-cerebral resuscitation, and reperfusion injury suggest that there may be a therapeutic role for magnesium in these conditions in the future.

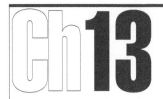

Colloids

Robert J. Murtaugh

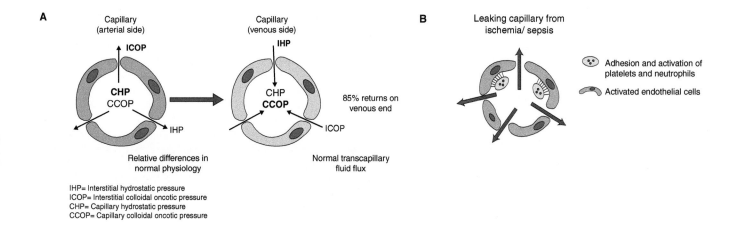

A

Capillary (arterial side)

ICOP

CHP
CCOP

IHP

Relative differences in normal physiology

Capillary (venous side)

IHP

CHP
CCOP

ICOP

85% returns on venous end

Normal transcapillary fluid flux

IHP= Interstitial hydrostatic pressure
ICOP= Interstitial colloidal oncotic pressure
CHP= Capillary hydrostatic pressure
CCOP= Capillary colloidal oncotic pressure

B

Leaking capillary from ischemia/ sepsis

Adhesion and activation of platelets and neutrophils

Activated endothelial cells

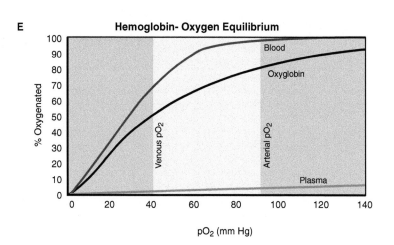

C

Colloids

Vasoconstriction

Tachycardia

Compensation for shock

Resuscitation with colloids

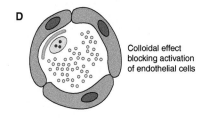

D

Colloidal effect blocking activation of endothelial cells

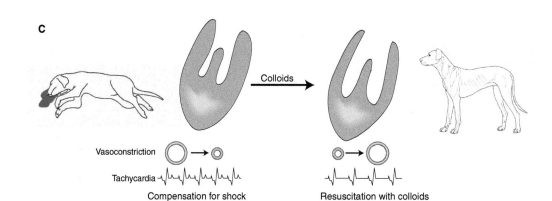

E

Hemoglobin- Oxygen Equilibrium

% Oxygenated

Blood

Oxyglobin

Venous pO$_2$

Arterial pO$_2$

Plasma

pO$_2$ (mm Hg)

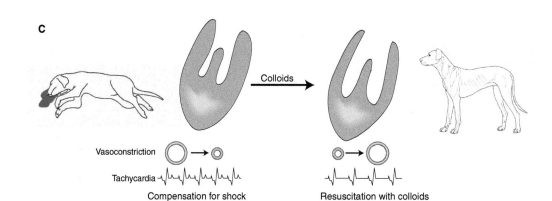

The extracellular fluid space is composed of the interstitial, transcellular, and plasma fluid compartments. The plasma and interstitial fluid compartments contain protein components, largely albumin, in solution. These protein fractions exert influence on the transcapillary movement of water and electrolytes (**Part A**). Plasma and interstitial fluid proteins are high-molecular-weight substances (>60 kd) that under normal physiological conditions are restricted by size and electrical charge from migrating through capillary endothelial pores. These protein fractions exert osmotic effects on transcapillary fluid fluxes that balance the effects of hydrostatic forces (see **Part A**). This osmotic effect is termed *colloidal oncotic pressure* (COP) and can be measured in blood with the use of a colloid osmometer. The measurement of serum albumin concentration and total serum solids by a refractometer can be used to estimate plasma COP.

Malnutrition and chronic diseases associated with decreased production or increased loss of plasma proteins such as albumin cause diminished plasma and interstitial oncotic pressures, resulting in altered transcapillary fluid dynamics (see **Part A**). This can lead to the development of pulmonary or peripheral edema, ascites, and pleural effusion, resulting in hypovolemia and organ dysfunction. Additionally, many acute disease processes such as pancreatitis or sepsis can result in activation of inflammatory processes that alter capillary endothelial integrity. This causes "capillary leak" and a loss of plasma proteins into the interstitial fluid (see **Part B**). The plasma COP is diminished in these instances, which further exacerbates the potential for hypovolemia and organ dysfunction in the patient, owing to altered transcapillary forces (see **Part A**).

The maintenance of COP can be key to the successful resuscitation and management of critically ill patients with acute or chronic disease processes. The use of plasma transfusion is an approach to consider for restoration and maintenance of COP. The limited availability and expense associated with these products has led to the development of synthetic colloid solutions [dextrans, hydroxyethyl starch (HES)] for the treatment of these conditions. Compared to plasma, these plasma substitutes have advantages, including elimination of the risk for transfusion-related disease transmission, ready availability, ease of room-temperature storage, and a long shelf life. The rapid infusion of these synthetic colloid solutions also can be used for the resuscitation of patients in shock. The rapid increase in plasma COP associated with IV bolus administration of dextrans or HES (hetastarch) causes a transcapillary shift of fluid into the vascular space, reversing hypovolemic shock (**Part C**).

Description of Synthetic Colloids

HES and dextran 70 are synthetic colloids composed of carbohydrate polymers with mean molecular masses of approximately 70 kd. Both colloids are packaged as 6% solutions in 0.9% saline solution. The intrinsic COP of these solutions causes an increase in intravascular volume through resorption of interstitial fluid in the capillary beds (see **Part A**). A comparable intravascular volume expansion with infusion of isotonic crystalloids such as LRS would require fourfold larger doses. Crystalloids lack intrinsic COP and disperse rapidly over the intravascular and interstitial fluid spaces. The effects on COP and intravascular volume expansion are measurable for up to 24 hours following IV bolus administration of HES and dextran 70.

All synthetic colloids have some influence on hemostatic mechanisms following administration. An inhibition of plasma clotting factor activity and platelet function is observed for approximately 24 hours after administration of HES and dextran 70. These effects are usually of minimal clinical significance. These hemostatic properties of synthetic colloids are potentially advantageous in patients at risk for disseminated intravascular coagulation due to compromised microvascular circulation.

The enhancement of microvascular circulation with administration of synthetic colloids has been known for many years, but only recently have the mechanisms for this effect been identified. Sepsis, for example, is associated with markedly increased plasma concentrations of adhesion molecules that indicate neutrophil and endothelial cell activation. Continuous IV infusion therapy with HES limits this process (see **Part D**). Xanthine oxidase release is decreased with HES administration following splanchnic ischemia-reperfusion, resulting in decreased multiple-organ system injury.

Treatment

The clinical uses for synthetic colloids span the spectrum of acute resuscitation of patients with shock, to chronic maintenance of COP for preservation of microvascular circulation in critically ill patients. In patients with hypotension and hypovolemia, dextran 70 and HES are administered routinely by IV bolus at doses of 5–20 mL/kg. The co-administration of hypertonic saline solution (7.5%) with synthetic colloids provides for a rapid (hypertonic saline) and sustained (colloid) resuscitation of hemodynamic parameters in patients with shock. The use of synthetic colloids for initial or continued resuscitation is indicated in hemodynamically unstable patients with hypoproteinemia (total serum solids <3.5 gm/dL or serum albumin concentration <2.5 gm/dL). As synthetic colloids "steal" from the interstitial fluid compartment to expand the intravascular fluid compartment, maintenance isotonic crystalloid administration is necessary to replace and replenish lost or shifted body fluids following acute resuscitation with colloids.

The preservation of COP has significance in the treatment of patients with acute injury or severe ongoing critical care needs. For example, a reduction of COP can aggravate brain edema and promote secondary brain injury following traumatic head injury. Dogs or cats with a critical illness or postoperative condition requiring intensive care that have COP values <14 mm Hg are at risk for development of tissue edema and organ system dysfunction. The COP of whole blood in healthy dogs and cats ranges from 18 to 25 mm Hg. The use of a continuous IV infusion of 20–40 mL of HES/kg/day can increase the COP of critically ill dogs by 8–10 mm Hg. The goal of therapy in critically ill patients should be to maintain a whole blood COP of at least 15 mm Hg.

The Future: Hemoglobin-Based Oxygen Carriers

Hemoglobin-based oxygen carriers (HBOCs) have been developed from bovine and human blood as well as by recombinant techniques. These HBOCs are purified, polymerized hemoglobin solutions with colloidal properties similar to HES and dextran 70 along with the additional characteristic of providing oxygen carriage. One of these solutions (Oxyglobin, Biopure Corporation, Cambridge, Mass.) is approved for use in dogs. Oxyglobin can be stored at room temperature, has a 2-year shelf life, and can be administered through a standard IV administration set. Oxyglobin requires no blood-typing or cross-matching prior to administration. The oxyhemoglobin dissociation curve of Oxyglobin is shifted rightward in comparison to that of red blood cell hemoglobin, resulting in a lower affinity of the HBOC for oxygen and an improved off-loading of oxygen from Oxyglobin in the tissues (**Part E**). HBOC may supplant other colloids in the resuscitative treatment of patients with traumatic injury and other critical illness.

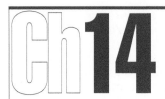

Analyzing Blood Gases

Steven Mensack

A   **Normal Arterial Blood Gas Values**

	Dog	Cat
pH	7.35 - 7.46	7.31 - 7.46
PCO_2	30.8 - 42.8	25.2 - 36.8
HCO_3^-	18.8 - 25.6	14.4 - 21.6
PO_2	90.9 - 103.3	95.4 - 108.2
BE_{ECF}	$^-4$ - $^+4$	$^-4$ - $^+4$

B

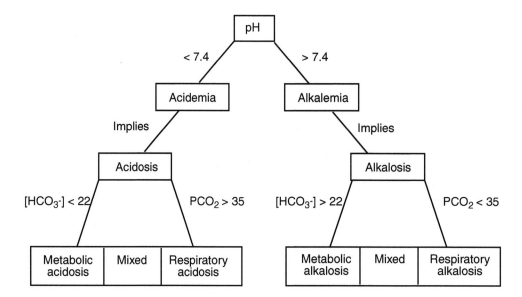

With the increased use of patient-side or point-of-care blood gas testing, thorough knowledge regarding the causes of and therapy for acid-base disturbances is necessary to extract the most information from these test results. Maintenance of a normal extracellular fluid environment is based on keeping the pH of this fluid within a narrow range (**Part A**). This range is maintained primarily by the buffering capacity of bicarbonate and carbon dioxide within the plasma, as illustrated by the equilibrium equation: $HCO_3^- + H^+ \leftrightarrow H_2CO_3 \leftrightarrow H_2O + CO_2$. Four primary acid-base disturbances are recognized: metabolic acidosis, metabolic alkalosis, respiratory acidosis, and respiratory alkalosis. This chapter focuses on how to analyze the data from a blood gas measurement and discusses mixed acid-base disturbances. Subsequent chapters focus on the primary acid-base disturbances.

pH

To understand acid-base chemistry, the clinician should be familiar with how to interpret the results of a blood gas analysis (**Part B**). There are 5 basic parameters on a blood gas analysis, figure B, pH, partial pressure of carbon dioxide (PCO_2), plasma bicarbonate (HCO_3^-), base excess, and partial pressure of oxygen (PO_2), which, while important, does not directly influence the assessment of acid-base status. The first step of this process is to evaluate the measured pH to identify if it is normal or if there is a primary disorder, an acidosis (decreased pH) or alkalosis (increased pH).

PCO_2 and HCO_3^-

Next, the HCO_3^- and plasma PCO_2 are evaluated in relation to the pH. As a general rule, if both the HCO_3^- and pH are decreased, then a primary metabolic acidosis exists; if the PCO_2 is increased while the pH is decreased, the primary disturbance is a respiratory acidosis; if the pH and HCO_3^- are increased, the primary disturbance is a metabolic alkalosis; and if the pH is increased and the PCO_2 is decreased, then the primary disturbance is a respiratory alkalosis. The next step is to determine if there is a normal compensatory response in the parameter opposite the primary disturbance (HCO_3^- for respiratory disturbances or PCO_2 for metabolic disturbances) or if a mixed acid-base disturbance exists. Compensatory changes occur to minimize the pH change associated with the primary disturbance. Again, there are several rules for evaluating the compensatory responses:

Metabolic acidosis—For each 1.0-mEq/L decrease in HCO_3^-, there should be a compensatory 0.7-mm Hg decrease in PCO_2.
Metabolic alkalosis—For each 1.0-mEq/L increase in HCO_3^-, there should be a compensatory 0.7-mm Hg increase in PCO_2.
Acute Respiratory acidosis—For each 1.0-mm Hg increase in PCO_2, there should be a compensatory 0.15-mEq/L increase in HCO_3^-. This change takes minutes to occur.
Chronic Respiratory acidosis—For each 1.0-mm Hg increase in PCO_2, there should be a compensatory 0.35-mEq/L increase in HCO_3^-. This change takes 2–5 days to occur.

Acute Respiratory alkalosis—For each 1.0-mm Hg decrease in PCO_2, there should be a compensatory 0.25-mEq/L decrease in HCO_3^-. This change takes minutes to occur.
Chronic Respiratory alkalosis—For each 1.0-mm Hg decrease in PCO_2, there should be a compensatory 0.55-mEq/L decrease in HCO_3^-. This change takes 2–5 days to occur.

Base Excess

The base excess is a calculated parameter on most blood gas analyses. It allows evaluation of the severity of a metabolic disturbance independent of compensatory respiratory changes. Base excess can range from -4 to $+4$ mmol/L in small animals and be considered normal. Patients with a positive base excess are alkalotic, and patients with a negative base excess (base deficit) are acidotic. As a guideline, a base excess or deficit $> \pm 10$ mmol/L denotes a significant metabolic acid-base disturbance that may be life-threatening, and corrective interventions are to be considered.

Mixed Acid-Base Disturbances

On occasion, it is possible for a patient to have >1 primary acid-base disturbance, a situation called a complex or mixed disorder. Mixed acid-base disorders can consist of an acidosis and an alkalosis, 2 acidoses, or 2 alkaloses. These types of disturbances are sometimes difficult to diagnose, but several guidelines may make it easier. The presence of a normal pH and an abnormal PCO_2 or HCO_3^-, or both, usually indicates a mixed disturbance. The exception to this rule is when a chronic respiratory alkalosis is present—in this situation, the metabolic compensatory response can return the pH to normal. A second guideline is that when the PCO_2 and HCO_3^- are changing in opposite directions, a mixed disturbance is often present. Finally, if the pH is changing in the opposite direction for a known primary disorder, then a mixed acid-base disorder is present. For example, an animal with known DKA with a pH of 7.5 has a mixed disturbance. When 2 primary disorders are suspected to be present, the use of the anion gap may help define these disturbances more completely. The anion gap is defined as the plasma cations ($Na^+ + K^+$) minus the plasma anions ($Cl^- + HCO_3^-$) and is normally 12–24 mEq/L in dogs and 13–27 mEq/L in cats. In general, an increase in the anion gap implies the accumulation of an organic acid (i.e., lactic acid), although alkalemia also can increase this value. Decreases in the anion gap are less common and may be due to hypoproteinemia (albumin is an unmeasured anion), respiratory acidosis, or severe hypernatremia.

As the final step of blood gas analysis, the findings should be evaluated against the clinical history and examination findings to ensure the blood gas results are consistent with the suspected etiology of the acid-base disorder. Then, a treatment plan should be devised.

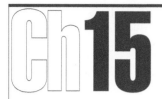

Ch15

Metabolic Acidosis

Steven Mensack

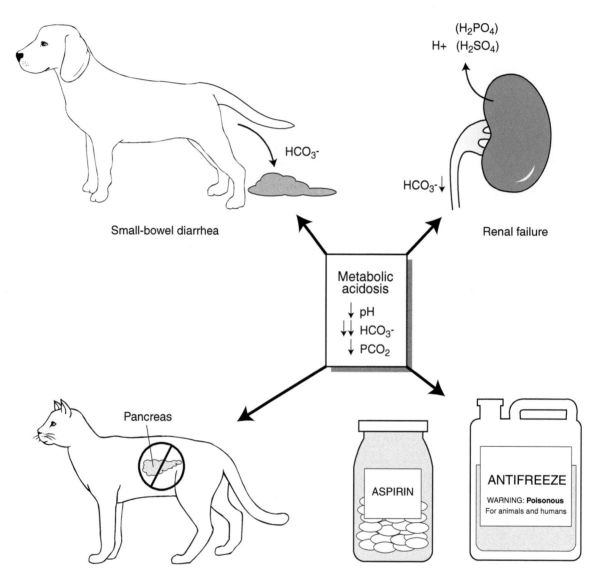

(H_2PO_4)

H+ (H_2SO_4)

HCO_3^-

Small-bowel diarrhea

$HCO_3^- \downarrow$

Renal failure

Metabolic
acidosis

$\downarrow$ pH

$\downarrow\downarrow$ HCO_3^-

$\downarrow$ PCO_2

Pancreas

ASPIRIN

ANTIFREEZE

WARNING: **Poisonous**
For animals and humans

Metabolic derangements: DKA, lactic acidosis

Toxic ingestion: aspirin, ethylene glycol

Metabolic acidosis is the most common acid-base abnormality encountered. It is present when there is a decrease in plasma HCO_3^- concentration, leading to a decrease in plasma pH. With intact ventilation, there is an adaptive decrease in the PCO_2 in plasma to mitigate the fall in pH. Recognizing and correcting metabolic acidosis is important, owing to the pathophysiological changes a decreased plasma pH can cause. Effects of acidosis include suppression of cardiac contractility, arteriolar vasodilatation, increased pulmonary vascular resistance, and increased susceptibility to ventricular arrhythmias. These effects are usually not noted until the plasma pH has decreased to <7.2.

Causes

There are 4 basic categories of causes for metabolic acidosis, and often more than 1 cause exists at a time. These categories are small-bowel diarrhea, metabolic derangements such as lactic acidosis and DKA, toxic ingestion of compounds such as ethylene glycol or aspirin, and renal disease (**Figure**).

Diarrhea
One cause of the development of metabolic acidosis is loss of bicarbonate in the GI tract from small-bowel diarrhea. In this situation, the increased amount of bicarbonate-rich fluid secreted into the small intestine overwhelms the colon's capacity for fluid reabsorption, and large amounts of bicarbonate are lost in the feces. Treatment of metabolic acidosis secondary to severe diarrhea involves identifying and eliminating the cause of the diarrhea. Rarely is acidosis strictly from diarrhea so severe that replacement bicarbonate therapy is warranted.

Metabolic Derangements
A second group of causes of metabolic acidosis includes several derangements in metabolism, most commonly lactic acidosis or DKA. Lactate is produced by most tissues as a product of anaerobic metabolism. Therefore, its production within a tissue greatly increases during conditions of decreased oxygen delivery. Conditions leading to the development of lactic acidosis include hypovolemic shock, septic shock, cardiogenic shock, seizure activity, strenuous exercise, anemia, and liver disease. The cause of the lactic acidosis should be identified and corrected. Tissue perfusion should be improved using aggressive fluid therapy if indicated or cardiac inotropes, or both. The use of sodium bicarbonate in lactic acidosis should be reserved for cases where the correction of the inciting condition may take time and the acidemia may be affecting cardiac function (pH < 7.2).

DKA occurs when there is unregulated diabetes mellitus. The lack of insulin and increase of counterregulatory hormones lead to the increased utilization of fatty acids and the increased production of the ketoacids. The mainstays of therapy to correct the acidosis associated with DKA are fluid therapy and insulin. The insulin administered allows for the conversion of the ketoacids back to a usable form and allows for the regeneration of plasma HCO_3^-. Rarely is replacement sodium bicarbonate therapy needed, but can be considered when acidemia might lead to cardiovascular problems.

Toxic Ingestion
The third group of causes of metabolic acidosis involves the ingestion of either ethylene glycol (antifreeze) or acetylsalicylic acid (aspirin). With ethylene glycol ingestion, the formation of the metabolites glycolic acid and oxalic acid leads to the metabolic acidosis by liberating hydrogen ion (H^+) and thus consuming HCO_3^-. Therapy of the acidosis associated with ethylene glycol ingestion involves the administration of sodium bicarbonate. At the same time, therapy should be undertaken to prevent further absorption, to prevent the metabolism of ethylene glycol to its toxic metabolites, to enhance elimination of toxic metabolites, to correct electrolyte abnormalities, and to maintain renal function.

The ingestion of large quantities of aspirin can lead to metabolic acidosis. The metabolism of aspirin to salicylic acid does not cause a metabolic acidosis, but the salicylic acid interferes with cellular oxidative metabolism, leading to the production of lactic acid, ketoacids, and other organic acids. Therapy for aspirin toxicity involves taking steps to prevent further GI absorption, to enhance elimination, and to treat potential complications such as gastric ulceration. The measures taken to promote elimination also correct the metabolic acidosis. Administration of sodium bicarbonate enhances elimination through the mechanism of ion trapping: Alkalinization of blood and urine increases the proportion of the ionized form of the drug, causing more unionized drug to leave cells and enter the blood or urine where it is converted to the poorly diffusible ionized form. The administration of sodium bicarbonate should be avoided if a respiratory alkalosis is the primary acid-base disturbance present.

Renal Disease
The final cause of metabolic acidosis involves reduced acid excretion due to renal disease. Under normal conditions, the kidneys are responsible for reabsorbing all HCO_3^- that is filtered at the glomerulus and regenerating any HCO_3^- that cannot be metabolized back to bicarbonate once it has been used to buffer an acid. Regeneration of HCO_3^- involves the creation and excretion of ammonium ion (NH_4^+) in the renal tubule; a process called *renal acid excretion*. With chronic renal failure, the kidney tubule is unable to regenerate filtered bicarbonate effectively, leading to decreased plasma HCO_3^- and metabolic acidosis. Persistent acidosis associated with renal failure leads to loss of bone mass, as calcium carbonate is used as a primary source for new HCO_3^-. This compensatory mechanism makes the acidosis associated with renal failure usually mild (HCO_3^- rarely <15 mEq/L). Renal tubular acidosis, a condition where there is a specific defect in the handling of HCO_3^- in the tubule without problems in the remainder of the nephron, is rare in small animals. Therapy of acidosis associated with renal failure is often not necessary, but when needed, bicarbonate can be provided orally.

Therapy

The administration of sodium bicarbonate for the correction of metabolic acidosis requires careful consideration. Sodium bicarbonate should only be administered if 1) there is severe, life-threatening acidemia (pH <7.2, HCO_3^- <10); 2) the patient is able to ventilate adequately, as the administration of sodium bicarbonate will generate more carbon dioxide that must be eliminated by the lungs; or 3) HCO_3^- cannot be regenerated because it has been lost in the urine (renal failure) or feces (severe diarrhea). The amount of sodium bicarbonate needed to correct severe metabolic acidosis can be calculated:

$$HCO_3^-\ (\text{in mEq}) = 0.3 \times \textbf{Body weight (in kg)} \times (\textbf{Normal } HCO_3^- - \textbf{measured } HCO_3^-)$$

Half of the calculated amount can be administered IV over several hours and then additional blood gas analyses performed to assess the need for further supplementation. Potential complications of sodium bicarbonate therapy include hypernatremia, hypokalemia, hypocalcemia, the development of iatrogenic alkalosis, volume overload secondary to the large amount of sodium that may be administered, and paradoxical cerebrospinal fluid acidosis.

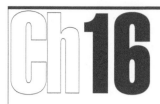

Respiratory Acidosis

Steven Mensack

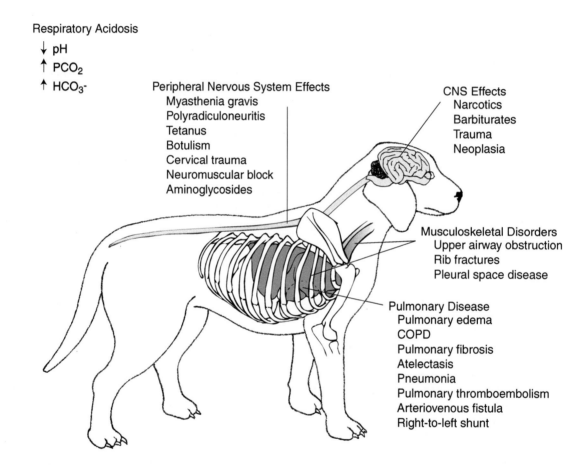

Respiratory Acidosis
↓ pH
↑ PCO_2
↑ HCO_3^-

Peripheral Nervous System Effects
Myasthenia gravis
Polyradiculoneuritis
Tetanus
Botulism
Cervical trauma
Neuromuscular block
Aminoglycosides

CNS Effects
Narcotics
Barbiturates
Trauma
Neoplasia

Musculoskeletal Disorders
Upper airway obstruction
Rib fractures
Pleural space disease

Pulmonary Disease
Pulmonary edema
COPD
Pulmonary fibrosis
Atelectasis
Pneumonia
Pulmonary thromboembolism
Arteriovenous fistula
Right-to-left shunt

Respiratory acidosis occurs when there is an increase in plasma PCO_2, leading to a decrease in plasma pH. It is important to be able to identify potential causes of acute respiratory acidosis immediately as these can be life-threatening. Disorders that can cause an acute onset of respiratory acidosis are usually associated with insufficient oxygenation of arterial blood (hypoxemia). This hypoxemia can be rapidly fatal and needs to be corrected immediately by securing an airway and ventilating for the patient if necessary. Other disorders slowly lead to respiratory acidosis with the development of a compensatory increase in plasma HCO_3^-. These chronic disorders usually are not immediately life-threatening as the patient has adapted to the hypoxemia present. Clinical signs associated with respiratory acidosis are likely due to the underlying disorder causing the respiratory problem rather than the retention of carbon dioxide itself, although cardiac arrhythmias, muscle weakness, paresthesia, papilledema, stupor, and coma can occur secondary to respiratory acidosis in people. There are 3 primary classes of disorders that lead to the increased PCO_2 seen with respiratory acidosis: problems with ventilation, problems with gas exchange, and disorders that lead to increased carbon dioxide production.

Causes

Hypoventilation
Ventilation refers to the movement of gas into and out of the lung. It involves the interplay of the respiratory centers in CNS, peripheral nerves, and thoracic musculoskeletal system in order to be effective. If the function of 1 of these systems is impaired, hypoventilation results. Causes of hypoventilation include CNS disorders associated with the action of drugs such as narcotic analgesics and barbiturates, cerebral trauma, and neoplasia; peripheral nervous system disorders such as myasthenia gravis, polyradiculoneuritis, tetanus, botulism, cervical trauma, and the use of drugs such as neuromuscular blocking agents, aminoglycosides, and organophosphates; and thoracic musculoskeletal disorders such as upper-airway obstruction, rib fractures, and pleural space diseases (pneumothorax, hemothorax, pyothorax, diaphragmatic hernia with abdominal contents displaced into the thorax) (**Figure**). A final cause of hypoventilation that should not be overlooked is iatrogenic hypoventilation in a patient receiving mechanical ventilation.

Gas-Exchange Disorders
Pulmonary gas exchange involves the movement of oxygen from the alveolus into the blood and the movement of carbon dioxide from the blood into the alveolus. Three categories of diseases can affect gas exchange: diffusion impairment, pulmonary ventilation-diffusion (V/Q) mismatch, and intrapulmonary or intracardiac shunt. Diffusion impairment occurs when equilibrium cannot occur between alveolar gas and pulmonary capillary blood because of a thickened alveolar wall or decreased contact time of blood with gas in the alveolus. Pulmonary fibrosis, chronic obstructive pulmonary disease (COPD), and pulmonary edema of any etiology are causes of diffusion impairment. V/Q mismatch occurs under conditions where areas of the lungs are receiving adequate fresh gas from the environment but blood flow is inadequate to effect gas exchange (V/Q >1) or when areas of the lungs are not receiving fresh gas from the environment but are receiving a normal supply of fresh blood for gas exchange (V/Q <1). Atelectasis, alveolar pneumonia, pulmonary edema, and pulmonary thromboembolism can cause V/Q mismatching. Shunts are an extreme form of V/Q mismatch where blood in the pulmonary circulation totally bypasses ventilated lung before returning to the systemic circulation.

Lung lobe consolidation, arteriovenous fistulas, and right-to-left intracardiac shunts are causes of these shunts.

Increased Carbon Dioxide Production
Conditions that increase the production of carbon dioxide include fever, physical activity, anxiety, and hyperthyroidism. The increased production of carbon dioxide by itself does not lead to respiratory acidosis in a patient with healthy lungs but can contribute to the condition if a concomitant problem with hypoventilation or gas exchange exists.

Compensation

Compensatory changes in HCO_3^- secondary to respiratory acidosis normally occur in 2 phases.

Acute Compensatory Response
The first phase occurs within 10–15 minutes of the onset of the increase in PCO_2. Based on the equilibrium equation ($H_2O + CO_2 \leftrightarrow H_2CO_3 \leftrightarrow HCO_3^- + H^+$), the acid ($H^+$) generated during respiratory acidosis cannot be buffered by the existing plasma HCO_3^-. Therefore, H^+ is primarily buffered intracellularly by hemoglobin, phosphate, or lactate. Of the intracellular buffers, only the buffering effect of hemoglobin leads to the creation of HCO_3^-, which is then returned to the plasma. Since only a portion of the H^+ that is buffered leads to the creation of HCO_3^-, the acute compensatory response to respiratory acidosis is not as strong as the chronic response.

Chronic Compensatory Response
The second phase of compensatory adaptation to respiratory acidosis normally takes 2–5 days to become fully effective. During this time, the kidneys adapt to the more acidic environment through net acid excretion and the generation of new HCO_3^-. At the same time, the renal reabsorptive capacity for HCO_3^- is increased. This increased capacity allows the new, higher rate of $[HCO_3^-]$ reclamation and regeneration to be maintained. This increased reabsorption of HCO_3^- is associated with an increased excretion of chloride ion (Cl^-) in the kidney; thus, hypochloremia commonly exists with chronic respiratory acidosis.

Therapy

Treatment of respiratory acidosis should be aimed primarily at identifying and relieving the underlying cause. In acute situations, airway management by tracheal intubation or tracheostomy, thoracocentesis, or reversal of narcotic analgesics may prove curative. Supplemental oxygen administration is usually of benefit since respiratory acidosis normally is accompanied by hypoxemia. In severe life-threatening situations, mechanical ventilation may be necessary while the underlying cause is remedied.

Management of chronic respiratory acidosis requires several steps. The underlying cause should be sought and appropriate treatment instituted. Supplemental oxygen also may be of benefit but should be used judiciously since hypoxemia may be driving ventilation by the time the patient is evaluated.

Overzealous use of oxygen may decrease this hypoxic drive, leading to worsening hypoventilation and carbon dioxide retention. If indicated, mechanical ventilation should be provided. Correction of the compensation for chronic respiratory acidosis does not require bicarbonate therapy. Instead, parenteral administration of fluids that contain adequate amounts of chloride help resolve the acidosis. This allows the kidneys to reabsorb chloride preferentially and excrete the additional HCO_3^- retained during the acidotic state.

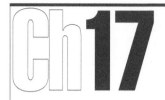

Metabolic Alkalosis

Steven Mensack

Metabolic Alkalosis

- ↑ pH
- ↑↑ HCO₃⁻
- ↑ PCO₂

Contraction Alkalosis

- Development of ↑HCO₃⁻
- Loss of H⁺ and water in vomitus
- Decreased vascular volume → ↑Na⁺ resorption
- Increased intravascular [HCO₃⁻]⁻ through renal mechanisms

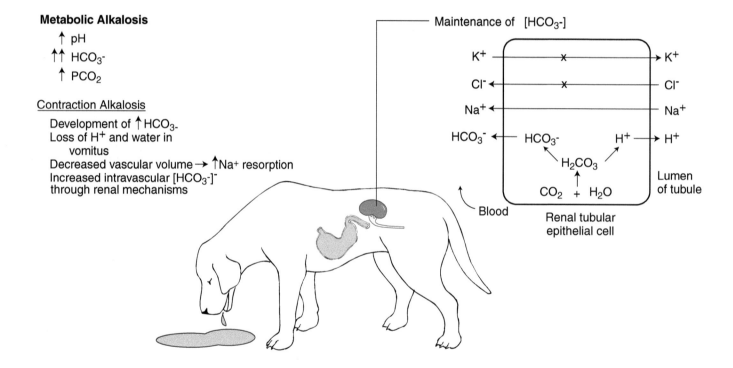

Metabolic Alkalosis

Metabolic alkalosis results from disease processes that cause an increase in the plasma bicarbonate [HCO_3^-], leading to an increase in plasma pH. In patients with an intact ventilatory system, there is resultant compensatory hypoventilation, which raises arterial PCO_2 and mitigates the rise in plasma pH. Recognizing and correcting metabolic alkalosis is important due to the pathophysiological changes an increased [HCO_3^-] can cause. Metabolic alkalosis is often accompanied by hypokalemia. The adverse effects of metabolic alkalosis and hypokalemia include ventricular and supraventricular arrhythmias; decreased oxygen delivery due to both the compensatory hypoventilation and a decrease in the ability of hemoglobin to unload oxygen at the tissues; and neuromuscular disorders including agitation, lethargy, muscular weakness, stupor, muscular twitching, seizures, and coma.

Etiologies

The development of metabolic alkalosis involves the causative process that leads to the abnormal accumulation of HCO_3^- and the development of factors that are responsible for maintaining the degree of alkalemia. There are 4 main categories of causes for metabolic alkalosis: loss of gastric fluid, diuretic therapy, posthypercapnia, and a group of disorders known as volume-resistant metabolic alkaloses. Each of these causes can lead to the development of volume depletion, hypokalemia, and aldosterone excess by various methods. The presence of these factors acts to allow the kidney to reabsorb more HCO_3^-, leading to the maintenance of the metabolic alkalosis.

One cause of the development of metabolic alkalosis is the loss of gastric fluid from vomiting or nasogastric suctioning (**Figure**). In the normal stomach, hydrogen ions (H^+) are secreted into the lumen to acidify the gastric contents. In order to produce this H^+, HCO_3^- is also produced according to the reaction $CO_2 + H_2O \rightarrow H^+ + HCO_3^-$. The HCO_3^- produced is transported into the blood. With continued vomiting of gastric contents or nasogastric suctioning, the stimulus for continued acid secretion persists, thus adding large quantities of HCO_3^- to the plasma. The loss of gastric fluid rich in Na^+, water, and K^+ leads to the development of the maintenance factors of volume depletion, hypokalemia, and aldosterone release discussed previously.

The treatment of edema with furosemide (Lasix) or thiazide diuretics is a most common cause of metabolic alkalosis. These medications cause a diuresis of extracellular fluid that contains virtually no HCO_3^-. This leads to a condition called *contraction alkalosis* where there is loss of extracellular fluid around a fixed amount of HCO_3^-. By a variety of mechanisms, diuretic use leads to the maintenance factors of hypovolemia, hypokalemia, and aldosterone excess.

The compensation for respiratory acidosis is elevated plasma [HCO_3^-]. If a patient with chronic respiratory acidosis is mechanically ventilated, and PCO_2 is rapidly reduced to normal, there is no immediate effect on [HCO_3^-]. The patient now has a high [HCO_3^-] and a normal PCO_2; by definition, a metabolic alkalosis exists. This condition is most commonly observed in patients with chronic pulmonary diseases that decompensate acutely requiring ventilatory support.

A group of disorders known as volume-resistant metabolic alkaloses can directly cause metabolic alkalosis that does not resolve with chloride-containing fluid therapy. These disorders include hyperaldosteronism, hyperadrenocorticism, and severe potassium deficiency. Although hyperadrenocorticism and severe potassium deficiency are commonly seen in dogs and cats, the metabolic alkalosis associated with these conditions is rarely considered.

Therapy

Treatment of metabolic alkalosis should be aimed at identifying and correcting the underlying cause(s). However, metabolic alkalosis can persist even with resolution of the underlying cause because factors that help maintain this condition are present. Volume depletion usually is treated by giving sodium and chloride–containing solutions IV. These solutions include normal saline solution (0.9% NaCl), Ringer's solution, and Normosol-R. Hypokalemia is repaired with potassium supplementation either within the IV fluids or by increasing the oral intake of food (if mild hypokalemia is present). The aldosterone excess in volume-responsive metabolic alkalosis is secondary to volume depletion. It self-corrects when volume is restored. With the underlying cause and maintenance factors removed, over a period of days the kidneys will excrete excess HCO_3^- and return plasma [HCO_3^-] to normal.

Respiratory Alkalosis

Steven Mensack

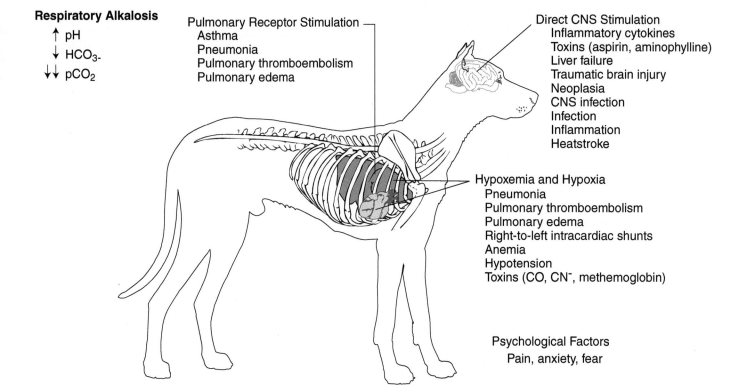

Respiratory Alkalosis
- ↑ pH
- ↓ HCO_3^-
- ↓↓ pCO_2

Pulmonary Receptor Stimulation
Asthma
Pneumonia
Pulmonary thromboembolism
Pulmonary edema

Direct CNS Stimulation
Inflammatory cytokines
Toxins (aspirin, aminophylline)
Liver failure
Traumatic brain injury
Neoplasia
CNS infection
Infection
Inflammation
Heatstroke

Hypoxemia and Hypoxia
Pneumonia
Pulmonary thromboembolism
Pulmonary edema
Right-to-left intracardiac shunts
Anemia
Hypotension
Toxins (CO, CN⁻, methemoglobin)

Psychological Factors
Pain, anxiety, fear

Respiratory alkalosis is the least commonly recognized acid-base derangement. This disorder is characterized by an increased pH, a primary decrease in PCO_2, and an adaptive decrease in HCO_3^-. Clinical signs due to respiratory alkalosis have not been observed in small animals. The presence of a disease process associated with respiratory alkalosis along with physical examination findings and blood gas analysis results confirming the acid-base disorder are needed to make the diagnosis.

Causes

Respiratory alkalosis occurs secondary to an increase in ventilatory drive. There are 4 classes of stimuli that can lead to this increase: arterial hypoxemia or tissue hypoxia, direct stimulation of pulmonary mechanoreceptors or chemoreceptors, direct stimulation of the CNS respiratory center, and psychological factors (**Figure**).

Arterial hypoxemia leads to stimulation of the CNS respiratory centers. The hypoxemic stimulation to ventilation increases linearly as arterial oxygen saturation (SaO_2) falls. Because of the sigmoid shape of the hemoglobin saturation curve, most patients have adequate saturation (>90%) as long as arterial oxygen partial pressure (PaO_2) is >60 mm Hg. Once PaO_2 falls below this level, SaO_2 declines markedly and hypoxemic drive becomes increasingly stronger. The increased ventilation attempts to increase PaO_2 but in the process, lowers PCO_2. Conditions leading to hypoxemia include pneumonia, pulmonary thromboembolism, pulmonary edema, right-to-left cardiac shunts, and congestive heart failure.

Other conditions cause tissue hypoxia without producing arterial hypoxemia. These hypoxic conditions also lead to increased ventilatory drive and subsequent decreases in PCO_2. Conditions leading to tissue hypoxia include severe anemia, hypotension, cyanide toxicity, methemoglobinemia, and carbon monoxide poisoning.

Within the walls of the alveoli and airways are stretch and irritant receptors (mechanoreceptors and chemoreceptors, respectively). When stimulated, these receptors lead to increased ventilation and can cause hyperventilation even if PaO_2 and oxygen delivery are normal. Pulmonary conditions that can stimulate these receptors include asthma, smoke inhalation, pneumonia, pulmonary thromboembolism, and pulmonary edema of any etiology.

Certain blood-borne compounds or CNS diseases have the ability to directly stimulate the medullary respiratory center, causing hyperventilation. These hematogenous compounds include inflammatory cytokines released during sepsis or CNS infection, toxic metabolites of aspirin or methylxanthine bronchodilators (aminophylline), and nitrogenous wastes liberated during hepatic failure. Central neurological disease associated with the development of respiratory alkalosis includes trauma, neoplasia, infection, cerebrovascular accidents, and inflammatory diseases such as granulomatous meningo-encephalitis (GME). Heatstroke also can lead to CNS-mediated hyperventilation.

The psychological factors of pain, anxiety, and fear can lead to hyperventilation in small animals.

Compensatory Response

Compensatory changes in HCO_3^- secondary to respiratory alkalosis normally occur in 2 phases: acute and chronic. The first phase (acute compensatory response) occurs within 10–15 minutes of the onset of the decrease in PCO_2. Based on the equilibrium equation $H_2O + CO_2 \leftrightarrow H_2CO_3 \leftrightarrow HCO_3^- + H^+$, the acid ($H^+$) needed during respiratory alkalosis cannot be created from existing plasma carbon dioxide since the equilibrium is shifted toward the production of carbon dioxide. Therefore, H^+ is contributed primarily from intracellular stores of proteins, phosphate, or lactate. This H^+ combines with existing plasma HCO_3^-, leading to a decrease in its plasma concentration. At the same time, potassium moves into cells, leading to a decrease in plasma K^+ concentrations. The acute compensatory response to respiratory alkalosis is not as strong as the chronic response.

The second phase of compensatory adaptation to respiratory alkalosis (chronic compensatory response) normally takes 2–5 days to become fully effective. During this time, the kidneys adapt to the more alkalotic environment through a decrease in net acid excretion. The retained H^+ further reduces plasma HCO_3^- and replaces the H^+ used for buffering in the acute period.

Therapy

Treatment of respiratory alkalosis should be aimed at identifying and correcting the underlying cause(s). In and of itself, hypocapnia is not dangerous in most situations, and no attempt is usually made to directly raise PCO_2. In the presence of traumatic brain injury, low PCO_2 can lead to excessive cerebral vasoconstriction and cerebral ischemia. In this situation, there may be benefit to correcting the hypocapnia. Hypoxemia, if present, should be ameliorated by providing supplemental oxygen. Pain, anxiety, or fear should be rectified using analgesics, tranquilizers, sedatives, or environmental modification.

Ch 19

Oxygen Therapy and Toxicity

Ann Marie Manning

A Causes of Hypoxemia

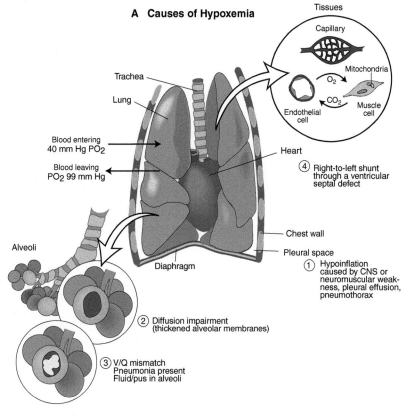

Tissues

Capillary

Mitochondria

O_2

CO_2

Endothelial cell

Muscle cell

Trachea

Lung

Blood entering 40 mm Hg PO_2

Blood leaving PO_2 99 mm Hg

Heart

④ Right-to-left shunt through a ventricular septal defect

Chest wall

Pleural space

Alveoli

Diaphragm

① Hypoinflation caused by CNS or neuromuscular weakness, pleural effusion, pneumothorax

② Diffusion impairment (thickened alveolar membranes)

③ V/Q mismatch Pneumonia present Fluid/pus in alveoli

B

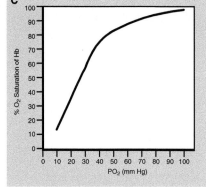

Target FIO2	Device	Oxygen Flow (L/min)
0.21-0.45	Nasal cannula	1-6
0.35-0.55	Facial mask	6-10
0.40-0.50	Oxygen cage	
0.50-0.90	Reservoir mask	5-15
0.50-1.00	Continuous positive-pressure airway	10-15

C

PO2 (mmHg)	% Saturation of Hb
100	97.5
90	96.5
80	94.5
70	92.5
60	89
50	83.5
40	75
30	57
20	35
10	13.5

D

O_2 → OO^- → H_2O_2 → OH^- (most potent oxygen free radical)

superoxide dismutase

lipid membrane

catalase

glutathione peroxidase ← selenium

H_2O H_2O

E Pathophysiology of Pulmonary Oxygen Toxicity

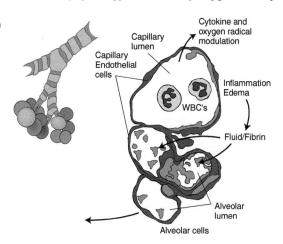

Cytokine and oxygen radical modulation

Capillary lumen

Capillary Endothelial cells

Inflammation Edema

WBC's

Fluid/Fibrin

Alveolar lumen

Alveolar cells

Oxygen supplementation increases the oxygen content of blood, improves tissue delivery of oxygen, and increases the PO_2, thereby increasing the distance through which oxygen diffuses into tissues. The administration of oxygen may improve the function of oxygen dependent cellular systems such as the cytochrome P_{450} system, nitric oxide synthase, and host defense systems. Given the important contributions supplemental oxygen can make, it is no wonder that oxygen is one of the most common drugs administered in the intensive care setting.

Physiology of Oxygenation

The important steps of oxygenation are oxygen uptake, diffusion, delivery, and metabolism. Oxygen uptake occurs with extraction of oxygen from the environment during respiration followed by movement of oxygen into the lungs, which serve as part of the delivery system. A pressure gradient between alveolar air (PO_2 99 mm Hg) and pulmonary capillary blood (PaO_2 40 mm Hg) provides the force for movement of oxygen across the respiratory membrane (surfactant, alveolar epithelium, and pulmonary capillary wall) into the systemic arterial blood where oxygen is bound with hemoglobin (Hb) (**Part A**). When blood reaches the tissue capillaries, oxygen diffuses down a gradient into mitochondria of interstitial cells. Eighty percent to 90% of the total oxygen is consumed by the mitochondria to produce energy in the process of oxidative phosphorylation.

Hemoglobin

Each Hb molecule reversibly binds 4 molecules of oxygen, and each fully saturated Hb molecule can transport 1.36 mL of oxygen. *Arterial oxygen content* (CaO_2) is the sum of oxygen dissolved in plasma plus oxygen bound to Hb.

$$CaO_2 = (Hb \times 1.36 \times SaO_2) + (PaO_2 \times 0.0031)$$

Oxygen dissolved in plasma is insignificant and is not important in oxygen transport unless cardiac output is substantially increased as in the case of severe anemia, or in hyperbaric oxygen therapy.

$$\textbf{Total oxygen delivery } (DO_2) = CaO_2 \times \textbf{cardiac output}$$

When the oxygen supply is adequate, oxygen consumption is a function of the metabolic rate. It is proposed that organ damage in critical illness is due to inadequate oxygen delivery and the level of tissue oxygen extraction not meeting metabolic demands. When oxygen supply fails to meet tissue demands, anaerobic metabolism takes over and lactic acid is produced.

Indications for Oxygen Therapy

Hypoxemia occurs in the presence of normal blood flow with decreased oxygen saturation (SaO_2), resulting in inadequate delivery of oxygen from the lungs to the blood. Hypoxemia can be caused by the following: 1) decreased fraction of inspired oxygen (FIO_2) (high altitudes, anesthetic accident), 2) alveolar hypoventilation where carbon dioxide displaces oxygen in poorly ventilated alveoli, 3) diffusion impairment, 4) ventilation-perfusion (V/Q) mismatch, and 5) right-to-left shunt (see **Part A**). Hypoxemia caused by low FIO_2 can be corrected by oxygen administration. Administration of oxygen during alveolar hypoventilation will provide temporary relief, but mechanical ventilation is optimal. Hypoxemia caused by right-to-left shunt will not respond to oxygen administration.

Anemic hypoxia occurs when inadequate Hb is available to transport a sufficient supply of oxygen for metabolism or when nonfunctional Hb such as methemoglobin (metHb) or carboxyhemoglobin (HbCO) is present. Supplemental oxygen administration is minimally helpful under these circumstances.

Stagnant hypoxia results from low blood flow and inadequate delivery of oxygen to the tissues. Hypovolemia secondary to intravascular dehydration or hemorrhage and low cardiac output states such as cardiogenic shock are examples of stagnant hypoxia. This form of hypoxia will respond to oxygen administration in conjunction with treatment of the underlying problem.

Modes and Techniques of Oxygen Delivery

A number of devices are available for oxygen delivery and the method chosen should be based on the FIO_2 desired and availability of equipment (**Part B**).

Monitoring Oxygen Therapy

Pulse oximetry is used to measure oxygen saturation or the percent of oxyhemoglobin (HbO_2) in the blood. **Part C**, the oxygen-hemoglobin dissociation curve, illustrates the relationship between the percent saturation of hemoglobin and PO_2. Pulse oximetry measures the functional saturation of Hb, not the fractional saturation. Fractional saturation can only be measured using a co-oximeter.

$$\textbf{Functional } O_2 \textbf{ saturation} = \frac{HbO_2}{HbO_2 + Hb}$$

Blood for intermittent *arterial blood gas* measurements can be taken from the femoral, dorsal metatarsal, or lingual artery to monitor PaO_2.

Oxygen Toxicity

When oxygen is administered at levels that exceed biotransformation and clearance, oxygen toxicity may result from the production of cytotoxic free oxygen radicals. Oxygen toxicity is a function of the duration of exposure and the PaO_2 rather than the FIO_2. With prolonged exposure to oxygen, antioxidant defense systems such as oxidase, superoxide dismutase, glutathione peroxidase, catalase, and free radical scavengers such as ascorbate, β-carotene, α-tocopherol, and *n*-acetylcysteine are overwhelmed and oxygen intermediates accumulate (**Part D**). Free oxygen radicals cause lipid peroxidation of cell membranes, with resultant loss of cell integrity. Oxidation of sulfhydryl groups alters enzyme function, damages protein structure, impairs transcription and replication of RNA, and causes defects of DNA cross-linking and nucleic acid damage.

The *pathophysiology* of pulmonary oxygen toxicity (**Part E**) can be separated into early and late stages. Initially, hyperoxia causes endothelial cell damage and destruction of alveolar lining cells, increasing microvascular permeability. Damage to the endothelium allows inflammatory precursors to enter the pulmonary interstitium, leading to alveolar edema, hemorrhage, and congestion. Polymorphonuclear cells adhere to the endothelial cells and generate chemotactic factors to attract more inflammatory cells. The early stages of pulmonary damage are characterized by proliferation of alveolar type I epithelial cells, a fibrin exudate, and a prominent alveolar membrane. In the late stages of oxygen toxicity, alveolar type I epithelial cells are lost, alveolar type II cells and fibroblasts proliferate, the basement membrane is denuded, and fibrosis results.

The *clinical signs* of oxygen toxicity include tachypnea, dyspnea, and a cough from tracheobronchitis secondary to decreased tracheal mucus velocity.

The *diagnosis* of oxygen toxicity is difficult and is based on an infiltrative lung pattern on radiographs, a worsening gas exchange (decreased PaO_2), and evidence of V/Q mismatch.

There is no effective *treatment* for oxygen toxicity; therefore, *prevention* is most important. The following steps are used to prevent toxicity. 1) Use a PaO_2 of 70 mm Hg as an end point for oxygen therapy. 2) Use the lowest FIO_2 possible to achieve a PaO_2 of 70 mm Hg. 3) Do not use an FIO_2 >0.6 for >24 hours. 4) Use positive end-expiratory pressure (PEEP) to help decrease the FIO_2 as necessary. The use of PEEP maximizes the PaO_2 at lower levels of FIO_2.

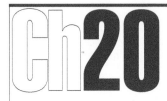

Transfusion Therapy

Elizabeth Rozanski

A **Feline Breeds and Blood Types**

Breed	Type A (%)
DLH/DSH	95
Abyssinian	80
Birman	80
British SH	40
Devon Rex	60
Himalayan	80
Persian	76
Others	80

B

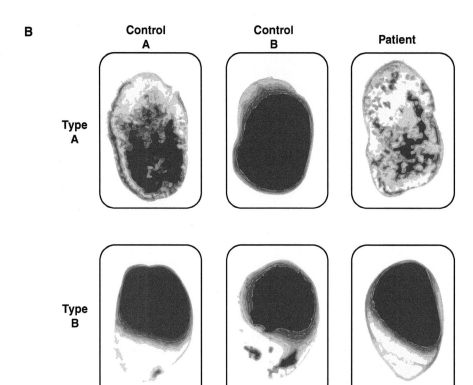

C

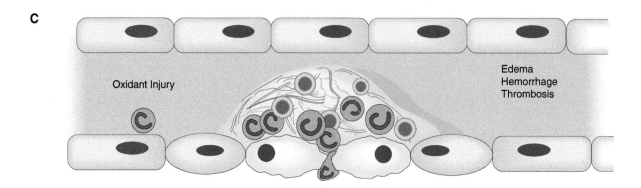

Over the past 10 to 15 years there has been a dramatic increase in both the availability and frequency of transfusions for animals. Most frequently, donated blood is divided into components to maximize the benefit from each unit of blood. The indications for blood transfusions include an increase in the oxygen-carrying capacity of the blood, replacement of missing/abnormal coagulation factors, protein replacement, and volume expansion.

Blood Groups and Types

Dogs have eight different blood groups. These are named dog erythrocyte antigens (DEA). Not all antigens are considered equally important in regards to their ability to trigger a transfusion reaction. DEA 1.1 is the most important antigen for dogs. Forty to fifty percent of dogs are positive for DEA 1.1. DEA 1.2 and DEA 7 may also play a role in triggering transfusion reactions. Transfusion of incompatible DEA 1.1 and 1.2 can result in hemolysis. Fortunately transfusion reactions are rare in dogs that have not previously been transfused. Dogs are unlikely to have preformed antibodies against other determinants. Blood type of both the recipient and the donor dog can be performed at a variety of laboratories and also with commercial blood typing cards.

The cat blood group system is made up of B and AB types. Cats differ from most other species because they have naturally-occurring alloantibodies to the other blood group even without previous transfusion. Type A is overwhelming the prevalent type in domestic mixed-breed cats in the United States (**Part A**). If a type A cat is given Type B, the transfusion will typically be hemolyzed within 48 hours. But if a Type B cat is given Type A blood, a fatal transfusion reaction will likely occur. Feline blood typing is available at reference laboratories. Commercial cards for blood typing cats have been developed (**Part B**). Ideally, all recipient cats should be typed prior to transfusion.

Blood Donors

Commercial or in-hospital blood banks provide a readily available source of blood or plasma for use in hospitalized patients. Pre-donation screening is strongly recommended for the donors. Typically, screening involves a physical examination, a complete blood count and chemistry profile. Species-specific screening for cats includes testing for feline leukemia and feline immunodeficiency viruses and for dogs, heartworm testing. In some geographic locations, testing for exposure to tick-borne diseases such as Erhlichia is also recommended.

The ideal feline donor is a large (more than 8–10 pounds) well-mannered adult cat. Most if not all cats require some sedation for donation. Feline blood donors should be carefully ausculted prior to sedation, as occult cardiomyopathies could contribute to morbidity or mortality for the donor cat. Approximately 50 ml of whole blood may be collected from a donor cat. Blood may be collected as frequently as every 4 weeks. The blood may be anticoagulated with heparin if it is to be used immediately, or with citrate-phosphate-dextrose-adenine (CPDA-1) for storage.

The canine blood donor is typically a large breed (more than 50 pounds) well-mannered adult dog. Retired racing greyhounds have been used extensively by the veterinary community as blood donors, due to their high hematocrit, large veins and docile natures. Approximately one unit (450 ml) may be collected from each donor. Generally canine blood is collected into bags containing CPDA-1.

Component Therapy

The different blood products that are available include fresh and stored whole blood, packed red blood cells, platelet-rich plasma, fresh frozen plasma, stored frozen plasma, cryoprecipate, and cryo-poor plasma. The most widely used components include packed red blood cells and fresh frozen plasma.

Fresh whole blood (FWB) contains red blood cells, platelets, leukocytes and plasma. Fresh whole blood is blood that is transfused within 12–24) hours of collection. The primary indications for transfusion with fresh whole blood include hemorrhage, thrombocytopenia with active hemorrhage, and lack of other available blood components. Stored whole blood may be stored for up to 35 days. The primary indication for the use of stored whole blood is hemorrhage or the lack of other readily available components.

Commonly individual units of canine whole blood are processed into components. The red cell portion of the unit is called packed red blood cells (pRBC). A unit of pRBC may be stored for 35 days at 4°C. The average hematocrit of a unit of pRBC is 70–80%. A unit of packed red cells is resuspended in saline (0.9%) prior to transfusion.

Plasma may be classified as fresh frozen plasma, stored plasma, platelet-rich plasma, cryoprecipate, or cryo-poor plasma depending on how the unit of whole blood is processed. The types of plasma differ in their presence and efficacy of the clotting factors. Fresh frozen plasma (FFP) is prepared by separating a unit of fresh whole blood within 6 hours of collection. FFP is a good source of all the clotting factors including V, VIII, and von Willebrands factor. FFP is stable for up to 1 year if stored at −40°C. After 1 year the more labile factor activity is diminished and the unit is termed stored plasma. Stored plasma has adequate amount of factors II, VII, IX, and X (the vitamin K dependent factors) and also albumin.

Platelet-rich plasma may be made by centrifugation of fresh whole bloods at lower than normal speeds (2,000xg vs 5000xg).

Cryoprecipitate may be prepared by thawing and centrifuging partially thawed fresh frozen plasma. Cryoprecipitate is very rich in clotting factors VIII, von Willebrands factor, and fibrinogen. Cryoprecipitate was initially created for use in people with congenital coagulopathies requiring multiple transfusions where volume overload with plasma products was a concern.

Transfusion Indications

The most frequent indication is to increase the oxygen-carrying capacity of the blood. The actual hematocrit at which a specific patient needs a transfusion is dependant on many factors. For example, a dog with pure red cell aplasia may be clinically normal with a hematocrit of 19%, while a dog with an acute hemoabdomen may be cardiovascularly unstable at a hematocrit of 28%. It is important to remember to transfuse the patient, not the hematocrit.

The amount of pRBC transfused depends upon the patient's size and hematocrit. On average, 5 ml of pRBCs/recipient body weight will increase the hematocrit by 10%. Packed red blood cells represent a significant intravascular volume load, so patients that are normovolumic or have pre-existing cardiovascular disease require careful monitoring during transfusion to prevent volume overload.

The indication for plasma transfusion is primarily replacement of clotting factors. Clotting factors may become diminished or dysfunctional via loss or dilution, consumption, production failure, or a combination of some or all of these reasons. Common clinical settings include disseminated intravascular coagulation, massive hemorrhage, and anticoagulant rodenticide poisoning (**Part C**). Careful assessment of the individual animal and its actual or anticipated deficiencies are essential for appropriate use of the specific type of plasma. In recent years, synthetic colloids have begun to replace plasma for volume expansion and albumin deficiency.

Transfusion reactions may range from mild (uticaria) to life-threatening (cardiovascular collapse and death). It is important to monitor the patient carefully for any signs of problems (vomiting, fever, hemoglobinuria/hemoglobinemia). Delayed transfusions may also occur due to the development of alloantibodies. Transfusions of both plasma and pRBC should be completed within 4 hours.

Pathophysiology of Pain

Ari Jutkowitz

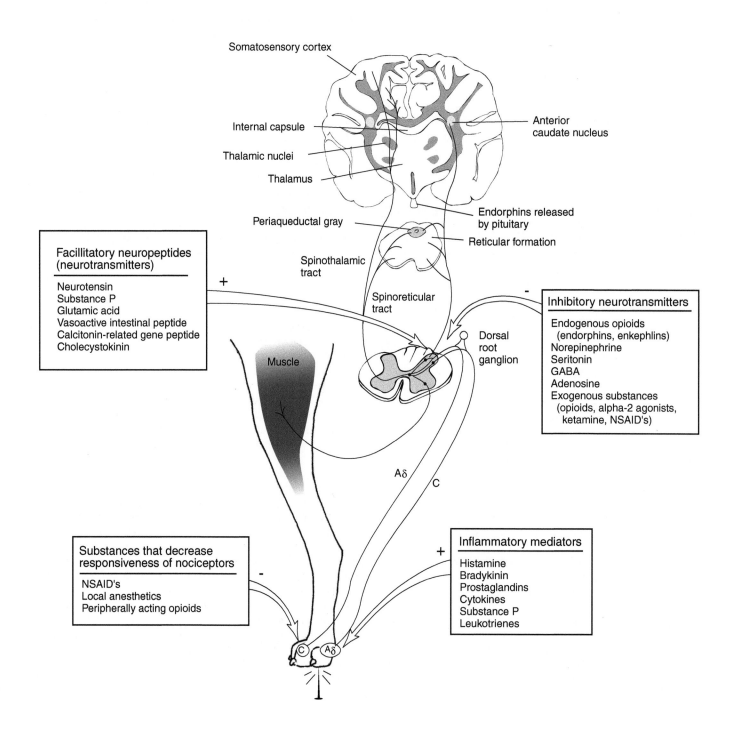

Pain is an individual experience derived from the complex interaction of sensory, emotional, environmental, and genetic factors. The nociceptive pathway accounts for how the location and extent of an injury are recognized, but other factors such as anxiety, fear, stress, and disruption of normal sleep cycles and family interactions also can affect perception of pain. The system that allows us to perceive pain is not a "hard-wired" system with a standard response to a given stimulus. Rather, pain pathways have a dynamic element so that prolonged painful stimuli result in long-term changes to the wiring of the nervous system, known as sensitization.

Physiologic pain resulting from a brief, noxious stimulus that causes relatively little damage to tissues can be viewed as a protective response. An example of this would be the pain of touching a hot stove. A more persistent pain results when inflammation, induced by mild tissue trauma, sensitizes nociceptors so that they respond to lower-intensity stimuli. This too serves a protective function, and the nociceptive system "resets" itself once the injury is healed. *Pathologic pain* resulting from chronic inflammatory processes like arthritis or cancer, or acute conditions like trauma or surgery, serves a less clear role in the well-being of the individual and should be treated whenever possible.

The Nociceptive Pathway

Nociceptors are generally the initial structures involved in the process of pain perception. They are sensory receptors that when activated by a stimulus capable of producing tissue damage, generate an impulse that is then transmitted along afferent fibers toward the spinal cord. The two main types of nociceptors are the *A delta* (mechano-heat) nociceptors, which respond to pressure and thermal injury, and the *C* (polymodal) nociceptors, which respond to heat, pressure, and chemical stimuli. Both *A delta* and *C* nociceptors are found in somatic structures, but *C* nociceptors alone are found in visceral organs. All nociceptors have an activation threshold, so that only stimuli of a high-enough intensity can result in the generation of an impulse.

The inflammatory response to injury results in release of inflammatory mediators (**Figure**) from macrophages, lymphocytes, and mast cells. These mediators contribute to the nociceptive process by directly stimulating nociceptors, by sensitizing receptors to the effects of other stimuli, and by prolonging the inflammatory response through vasodilation, chemotaxis, and edema. Neuropeptides (see **Figure**) released from afferent fibers cause changes in the excitability of nerve fibers, further release of inflammatory mediators, vasodilation, and plasma extravasation. The effect of the inflammatory response is sensitization, enhanced responsiveness of individual nociceptors to lower-intensity impulses. Additionally, silent nociceptors, which under normal circumstances do not respond to stimuli, are recruited into activity.

Afferent nerve fibers carry the impulse generated by the nociceptor toward the spinal cord. There are two major types of afferent fibers, *A delta* and *C*, that transmit nociceptive signals from their corresponding nociceptors. *A delta* fibers are small, myelinated fibers that transmit impulses very rapidly. These fibers are associated with "first pain," the initial sharp pain felt when an injury occurs. *C* fibers are unmyelinated fibers with a relatively slower rate of transmission, and these fibers become increasingly important with repeated stimulation. These are associated with "second pain," the dull, throbbing that follows an injury, and with the chronic pain of arthritis and other inflam-

matory conditions. *C* fibers are the only nociceptors in visceral structures, and their sparse distribution in these structures accounts for the poorly localizing character of visceral pain.

The dorsal horn of the spinal cord is the site where the afferent fibers terminate. Integration and processing of nociceptive input from all the various afferent fibers occur at this level. Noxious signals coming in from the periphery can be either transmitted on toward higher centers or suppressed here. Facilitation and inhibition are mediated by various neuropeptides (see **Figure**) that are stored in the dorsal root ganglion. The two main types of second-order neurons in the dorsal horn are nociceptor-specific neurons, which respond only to noxious stimuli, and wide dynamic range neurons (WDRN) which respond to both noxious and tactile stimuli.

WDRN windup is the process by which second-order neurons in the dorsal horn are sensitized following repeated noxious stimuli. The repetitive firing of *C* fibers results in continuous neurotransmitter release in the dorsal horn, enhancing the responses of second-order neurons so that they respond more vigorously and for a longer duration to subsequent stimuli. Although WDRNs normally do not signal pain in response to a tactile stimulus, following sensitization they may have an exaggerated response to low-intensity stimuli so even a light touch may be perceived as painful (hyperalgesia). Preventing WDRN windup and other sensitization mechanisms is the reason behind preemptive analgesia, the theory that analgesics should be administered before surgical pain is induced.

Following processing in the dorsal horn, the signal is then transmitted to higher centers by way of ipsilateral nociceptive pathways. The spinothalamic tract ascends to various nuclei in the thalamus, where the many nociceptive impulses are consolidated. From the thalamus, third-order neurons carry the noxious stimulus to the parietal (somatosensory) cortex where localization of pain takes place, and to the frontal lobe and cingulate cortex where motivational-affective or emotional responses to pain are mediated. The spinoreticular tract ascends from the spinal cord to the reticular formation in the brainstem, an area also involved in triggering affective responses to pain.

Descending modulation is the process by which nociception is inhibited. The periaqueductal gray is rich in opioid receptors, and also receives projections from a number of areas of the brain involved in antinociception. When stimulated, it initiates release of neurotransmitters that suppress further conduction at the level of the dorsal spinal cord horn.

Recognizing Pain in Animals Through Behavior

Behaviors in patients that indicate pain are not always as obvious as crying and holding up an injured paw. Other signs include tachycardia, tachypnea, salivation, aggression or submission, inappetence, dullness, and postural behaviors like reluctance to stand or lay down, guarding an injury, head droop, and the "prayer position" of abdominal pain. Many factors influence whether an animal will display behavioral signs of pain. Sick animals may lay quietly, too debilitated to show signs of pain. Young animals are more likely to show pain behaviors than are older animals, and dogs are more likely to demonstrate pain than cats. Certain breeds, like collies, may be more prone toward vocalizing when stressed or in pain. Because of the unreliability of behavioral indicators, simply knowing that an injury or illness has the potential to cause pain should be all we need to know before starting pain management.

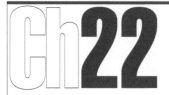

Analgesia I: Systemic

Justine A. Johnson

A Sites of Action of Analgesic Drugs

Sensory cortex — General anesthesia
Internal capsule — Dissociative anesthesia
Thalamus — Systemic opioids α2 agonists
Periaqueductal gray
Systemic opioids α2 agonists
Mesencephalon
Spinal nerve
Spinal local anesthesia
Spinal and systemic opioids
Acupuncture
α2 antagonists
Laminae of dorsal horn
Medulla
Dorsal root ganglion
Peripheral nerve
Local anesthetic wound infusion
Nociception
Local anesthetic nerve block
NSAIDs
Nursing care
Noxious stimulus
Lateral spinothalamic tract
Spinal cord

B Opiate Receptor — Action of Agonists

Receptor	Action
μ	Analgesia (spinal, supraspinal), respiratory depression, bradycardia, miosis, euphoria, emesis, ileus
κ	Sedation, analgesia, mild respiratory depression, miosis
σ	Excitement, dysphoria, tachycardia, tachypnea, mydriasis
δ	Analgesia, hypotension, bradycardia, respiratory depression, ileus
ε	Not well established

C Effects of Opioids and a2-Adrenergic Agonists at their Respective Receptors

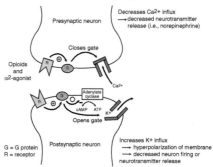

Presynaptic neuron — Decreases Ca2+ influx → decreased neurotransmitter release (i.e., norepinephrine)
Closes gate
Opioids and α2-agonist
Adenylate cyclase
cAMP ATP
Opens gate
G = G protein
R = receptor
Postsynaptic neuron
Increases K+ influx → hyperpolarization of membrane → decreased neuron firing or neurotransmitter release

E Commonly Used NSAIDs

NSAIDs	Dose	Comments
Acetaminophen	Dog: 15 mg/kg PO q8 hr. Do not give to cats	Not very effective for treatment of musculoskeletal pain unless combined with codeine; toxic to cats
Acetylsalicylic acid	Dog: 10-25 mg/kg PO q8 hr. Cat: 10mg/kg PO q72 hr	Only moderately effective for musculoskeletal pain, gastric irritation common, enteric coated tablets available; cats require careful dosing
Carprofen	Dog, Cat: 4.0 mg/kg IV, IM, SQ postsurgical, or 2.2 mg/kg PO q12 hr for chronic use	Weaker COX-1 inhibition than other NSAIDs, low GI toxicity, occasional liver toxicity
Etodolac	Dog: 10-15 mg/kg PO q24 hr	More COX-2 specific than most other NSAIDs, recommended for chronic therapy of pain associated with osteoarthritis
Ketoprofen	Dog, Cat: 2.0 mg/kg IV, IM, SC initially, then 0.5-1.0mg/kg q24 hr	Effective in management of postoperative pain, and can be used chronically in cats and dogs
Ketorolac	Dog: 0.3-0.5 mg/kg IV or IM postsurgical	Effective in management of postoperative pain, GI effects common, renal toxicity in compromised patients

D Effects of Commonly Used Opioid Analgesics

	Receptor Effects μ κ σ	Respiratory Depression	Bradycardia	Hypotension	Histamine Release	Emesis	Ileus / Constipation	Antitussive	Comments	Dosage
Pure agonist										
Morphine		+	+	+	+	+	+		Decreases oxygen consumption and myocardial work	Dog: 0.1-1.0 mg/kg IV, IM, SC q4-6 hr; epidural: 0.1 mg/kg IM,SC. Cat: 0.1 mg/kg q3-6hr IM,SC (dysphoria common)
Oxymorphone	+ +	+	+	+			+			Dog: 0.1-0.2 mg/kg IV, IM, SC q2-3 hr (auditory hypersensitivity common). Cat: 0.05-0.15 mg/kg IM,IV q2-4hr (excitement common)
Fentanyl	+ +	+	+	+	+		+	+	Very short duration of action unless transdermal patch or CRI	Dog: 25 mcg per 10 kg transdermal patch, q72 hr; 0.1-1.0 mg/kg/hr CRI IV. Cat: 25 mcg transdermal patch per cat, q96 hr
Meperidine	+ +	+		+						Dog: 5-10 mg/kg IV (very slowly), IM q2-4 hr PRN. Cat: 3-5 mg/kg IM, SQ q2-4 hr PRN
Codeine	+ +	+						+		Dog: 0.5-1.0 mg/kg PO q4-6 hr (if includes acetaminophen, do not exceed 15mg/kg acetaminophen)
Agonist / antagonist										
Butorphanol	- + +	+/-	+/-					+	May antagonize effects of pure agonists at μ-receptor while maintaining κ–mediated analgesia; ceiling effect to respiratory depression	Dog: 0.2-0.4 mg/kg IV, IM, SC q2-4 hr. Cat: 0.2-0.8 mg/kg IV, IM, SC q2-6 hr (May be used to reverse effects of pure μ agonists, while maintaining κ-mediated analgesia; ceiling effect to respiratory depression)
Pentozocine	- + +	+					+	+	Very short duration of action	Dog: 1.7-3.3 mg/kg IM q4 hr. Cat: 2.2-3.3 mg/kg IV, IM, SC q4 hr (dysphoria common)
Buprenorphine	+/-		+	+	+				Relatively long duration of action	Dog: 0.006-0.02 mg/kg IV, IM, SC q4-8 hr. Cat: 0.005-0.01 mg/kg IV, IM q4-8 hr
Naloxone	- - -									Dog, Cat: 0.0- 0.04 mg/kg IV, IM, SC q1-2 hr (as needed to reverse opiate effects)
Nalbuphine	- + -									Dog, Cat: 0.01-0.5 mg/kg IV, IM, SC q3-6hr (as needed to reverse opiate effects, use low end of dose in cats)

+ = Agonist
- = Antagonist
+/- = Partial agonist

There are multiple steps in the perception of pain. Peripheral nociceptors respond to noxious stimuli, and the impulse generated is transmitted along peripheral neurons to the dorsal horn of the spinal cord. Here the neurons synapse with neurons in the spinothalamic tract, which carry the impulse to the brain, resulting in the conscious recognition of pain. Analgesic techniques can be directed at any of these segments in the pain transmission pathway (**Part A**).

Painful stimuli and the psychological effects of pain perception can result in a complex cascade of physiological events including the recruitment of the sympathetic-adrenal and hypothalamic-pituitary axes. This "stress response" results in a hypermetabolic state. If this state is prolonged, it can result in lactic acidosis, the exhaustion of energy stores, impaired healing, GI ulcerations, and organ failures due to poor perfusion. Following thoracotomy, chest injuries, and thoracolumbar spinal procedures, pain associated with moving or expanding the thoracic cage can result in poor pulmonary function. Reduction of nociceptive input and pain perception through analgesic techniques can ameliorate the stress response and the effects of pain on pulmonary function.

Pre-emptive Analgesia

While general anesthesia prevents the conscious perception of pain during surgery, it does not stop nociceptive transmission or prevent the physiological effects of nociception. Tissue injury, including surgical wounds, can cause a hyperexcitable state, known as *windup,* in dorsal horn neurons. This phenomenon results in a prolongation or sensitization to pain that can persist beyond the end of surgery. Preemptive analgesia reduces the input from peripheral nerves during anesthesia and therefore, may reduce the amount of analgesic medications required during the postoperative period.

Analgesic Drugs

Narcotics

Opioid receptors are found in high density in the dorsal root ganglia and substantia gelatinosa of the spinal cord as well as the brain stem, thalamus, and cerebral cortex (**Part B**). The binding of opiate drugs to their receptors on neuron cell membranes causes activation of G proteins (**Part C**). The G proteins regulate ion channels and inhibit the activity of adenylate cyclase, the enzyme that catalyzes cAMP synthesis. The effect is to raise the threshold for neuron excitability and decrease the release of neurotransmitters. The pure opiate agonists generally act on μ and κ receptors, inducing analgesia and sedation. There is no ceiling effect to the pure agonists, so increasing doses induces greater analgesia; however the doses and usage of these drugs are limited by their side effects (**Part D**). Mixed agonist-antagonist opioids and partial agonist opioids have variable effects at the μ and κ receptors, but generally cause less dysphoria, sedation, and respiratory depression compared to pure agonists. Side effects of opiate analgesics, especially sedation and respiratory depression, often can be reversed by opiate antagonists such as naloxone and nalorphine.

α₂ Agonists

The stimulation of α₂-adrenergic receptors by their agonists (xylazine, detomidine, medetomidine) inhibits the transmission of painful stimuli at the level of spinal cord interneurons, resulting in spinal analgesia. The α₂ adrenoreceptors are also found in many of the same pain centers of the CNS as opioid receptors, and like opioid receptors, the α₂ adrenoreceptors activate G proteins, which mediate the opening of ion channels (see **Part C**). In the CNS, α₂ agonists act on presynaptic

adrenoreceptors, inhibiting the release of norepinephrine, a neurotransmitter that mediates arousal and pain. The α₂ adrenoreceptors also are located on the postsynaptic membrane in effector organs such as peripheral blood vessels and the heart, and their activation causes an increase in peripheral vascular resistance and blood pressure and can induce cardiac arrhythmias. However, the central sympatholytic effects are longer acting and result in systemic hypotension and bradycardia. The cardiovascular effects make these drugs unfit for use in hemodynamically unstable patients. The α₂-agonist effects can be reversed with the administration of yohimbine or atipamezole.

Dissociative Anesthetics

The dissociative cyclohexamine anesthetics (ketamine, tiletamine) provide somatic analgesia by interrupting nociceptive transmission in the CNS. They also inhibit the cortical recognition of painful stimuli by interrupting the transmission of impulses at the thalamoneocortical level. Their usefulness as analgesics is limited, however, because they also induce anesthesia.

Sedatives and Tranquilizers

Barbiturates, benzodiazepines, and phenothiazines often are utilized as part of an anesthetic regimen, or to quiet excitable patients. While these agents may participate in the treatment of pain by decreasing the patient's perception of or sensitivity to pain, they do not provide any direct analgesic effect.

NSAIDs

Nonsteroidal anti-inflammatory drugs (NSAIDs) inhibit cyclooxygenase (prostaglandin synthetase), which catalyzes the conversion of arachidonic acid to thromboxane, prostacyclin, and prostaglandins (PGE₂, PGF₂, PGD₂). These substances mediate inflammation, amplify nociceptive input and the transmission of nociceptive impulses along peripheral nerves, and increase the firing of central neurons and the release of neurotransmitters from spinal afferents. The use of NSAIDs near the time of injury can reduce the level of inflammation and the degree of nociceptive input associated with that injury, thus limiting the duration or dose of narcotic analgesics required.

There are 2 forms of cyclooxygenase. The negative side effects of NSAIDs are related to the inhibition of cyclooxygenase 1 (COX1), which catalyzes the production of prostaglandins that modulate renal blood flow, the synthesis of gastric mucus, and other physiological functions. Cyclooxygenase 2 (COX2) is activated in damaged or inflamed tissues and catalyzes the production of prostaglandins that sensitize nociceptors in areas of tissue injury. The ideal NSAID would inhibit COX2 with minimal effect on COX1. Several newer NSAIDs are considered to be more COX2 specific (carprofen, etodolac) (**Part E**). The use of NSAIDs is contraindicated in patients with poor perfusion states such as shock or hemorrhage, patients with existing renal disease, or patients already at risk for GI ulcers. Moderate or severe pulmonary disease may also be a contraindication, as inhibition of PGE₂ and prostacyclin may lead to constriction of bronchial and tracheal muscles.

Conclusion

Combination therapy including preoperative analgesics, adequate general anesthesia, local or regional analgesia (see Chapter 23) and post-operative combinations of NSAIDs and narcotics can be highly effective in limiting pain and suffering in the postoperative period. The appropriate combination should be selected for each individual patient based on the cardiopulmonary stability of the patient, the anticipated degree of postoperative pain, and coexisting medical conditions.

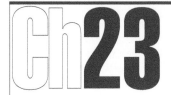

Analgesia II: Local and Regional Anesthesia

Justine A. Johnson

A   Local Anesthetics Block Sodium Channels Inhibiting Generation and Propagation of Action Potential

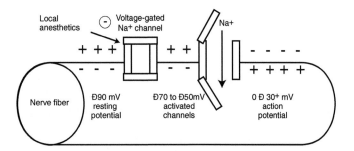

B

Block Location	Regional Analgesia
Brachial plexus	Elbow and points distal
Intercostal nerve	Thoracic wall ventral to injection site at each rib space injected (generally need to block 1-2 spaces to each side of wound)
Intrapleural block	Pleural surfaces of thorax
Caudal epidural	Hind legs, perineum, tail, caudal abdomen
Cranial epidural (via epidural catheter)	Hind legs, perinium, tail, caudal abdomen, cranial abdomen and part of thorax (blocks spinal segments 1-2 spaces cranial to tip of catheter)

C   Brachial Plexus Block

Following sterile prep of the site, a spinal needle is inserted medial to the shoulder joint and directed toward the costochondral junction and parallel to the vertebral column, to a depth of 3.5-7.5 cm (depemding on size of dog). Aspiration is performed to avoid injection into the blood vessel, then local anesthetic (4-6 ml/kg 2% lidocaine, or 1.5-2.0 ml/kg 0.5% bupivicaine) is injected slowly as the needle is withdrawn.

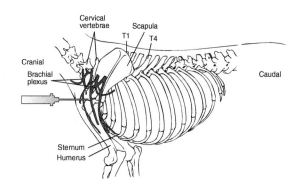

D   Intercostal Block

The nerve in the intercostal space of the thoracotomy incision is blocked, as well as two rib spaces cranial and caudal to the site. Local anesthetic (1.5 mg/kg of 0.5% bupivicaine divided into 5 doses, one for each nerve) is injected caudal to the rib, as far dorsally as possible.

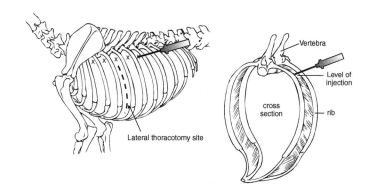

E   Intrapleural Injection

Local anesthetic 0.5mg/kg (cat) or 1.5mg/kg (dog) of 0.5% bupivicaine hydrochloride is instilled via thoracotomy tube (if present). Alternatively, an over-the-needle catheter is passed through an intercostal space and drug is instilled into thoracic cavity. Patient should be placed with affected side down after injection to allow gravity to deliver the drug where needed.

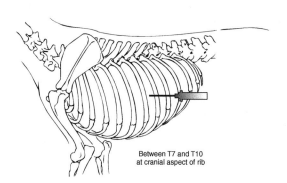

F   Caudal Epidural Injection

A surgical prep is performed over the lumbosacral junction. A spinal needle is passed through the supraspinous and interarcute ligaments at the lumbosacral junction (the L6-7 space can also be used, but penetration of the dura and subarachnoid injection are more likely). The reader is advised to refer to the references provided before attempting this procedure.

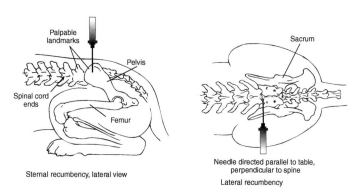

Systemic administration of narcotics and/or anti-inflammatories is the mainstay of analgesic therapy, but their use might be contraindicated in certain patients. The duration or dose of systemic analgesic agents can be minimized by applying a combination of systemic and nonsystemic methods of pain relief. For example, local and regional anesthesia prior to surgical procedures is an effective means of providing preemptive analgesia limiting the need for postoperative medications.

Local Nerve Blocks

The propagation of impulses along a nerve axon requires the generation of an action potential. The action potential is generated when voltage-gated sodium channels open in response to a stimulus, allowing sodium ions to enter the axon, making the membrane potential less negative (**Part A**). Local anesthetics bind to peripheral neuronal cell membranes and inhibit the opening of sodium channels, thus preventing the generation of the action potential. Small, sensory and autonomic fibers are affected first, followed by larger motor and proprioceptive fibers. The most common agents utilized in veterinary medicine are lidocaine and bupivacaine. Local anesthetics can be infused into tissue surrounding a wound area, can be used to block specific nerve activity to provide regional anesthesia, or can be injected into the epidural or subarachnoid space (**Parts B** to **E**). The duration of activity of local nerve blocks can be increased 15%–30% if the agent is mixed with epinephrine at 1:200,000. Toxic plasma levels of local anesthetics can occur in cases of inadvertent IV injection or absorption of high doses injected for local anesthesia. Cats are especially sensitive to local anesthetics and must be dosed carefully. Toxic effects include hypotension, AV block, arrhythmias, myocardial depression, and seizures or CNS depression if the agents cross the blood-brain barrier.

Epidural Analgesia

The administration of analgesic drugs into the epidural space can induce effective regional analgesia with limited systemic effects (**Part F**). Opiates, α_2 agonists, and local anesthetics are effective by this route. If administered preoperatively, epidural analgesia can limit the need for inhalant anesthesia and decrease the transmission of nociceptive stimuli during surgery, thus potentially decreasing postoperative pain. Epidural injection is most appropriate for procedures involving the hind limbs, perineal area, and tail; however, it can be effective for lower abdominal procedures as well. Epidural catheters can be used to provide prolonged administration of analgesics or to deliver analgesic more cranially for high abdominal or thoracic procedures. The use of epidural analgesia may decrease the pulmonary function changes associated with pain in patients undergoing thoracotomy. The combined use of local anesthetics and narcotic analgesics in the epidural space provides regional anesthesia during surgical procedures and analgesia in the postoperative period.

Opiates injected into the epidural space gain access to spinal receptors by diffusion across meninges, traveling along the perineurium of spinal nerves to the spinal cord, or absorption by spinal arteries. Compared to systemic administration, epidural administration of opiates provides prolonged analgesia. The duration of action of epidural opioids is longer for water-soluble drugs such as morphine, and short for lipid-soluble drugs such as fentanyl and buprenorphine. Epidural morphine can provide analgesia for up to 24 hours and oxymorphone for up to 10 hours. Epidural opioid administration can be associated with urine retention and pruritus. Preservatives found in some opioid preparations can be neurotoxic, so preservative-free products are recommended.

Local anesthetics in the epidural space block neuronal transmission at spinal nerves and within the spinal cord. Lidocaine induces spinal anesthesia for 60–90 minutes, whereas the effects of bupivacaine can last for up to 6 hours. Local anesthetics cause motor blockade, which usually lasts for a few hours but can persist, albeit rarely, for days to weeks. Cranial advance of the agent can cause complete spinal blockade, leading to intercostal and phrenic paralysis affecting respiratory function. Sympathetic blockade may cause hypotension, especially in hypovolemic patients.

Potential complications associated with epidural injections include infection (meningitis), hemorrhage (epidural, intrathecal), and spinal or nerve root trauma. The spinal cord ends cranial to L7 in large dogs, and more caudally in cats and smaller dogs. If the dura persists beyond L7, lumbosacral injection could introduce drug into the subarachnoid space. If this occurs, the drug is more likely to travel cranially, increasing the potential for side effects. If subarachnoid injection is suspected because of the size of the patient or the appearance of fluid in the spinal needle, the volume of drug should be decreased by 50%. Strict aseptic technique must be followed during epidural injection. Contraindications to epidural injection include septicemia, coagulopathy, local skin infection, and lumbosacral injury.

Other Techniques of Pain Management

Acupuncture

Acupuncture is the insertion of needles at specific points to produce physiological responses, including analgesia. Acupuncture sites contain increased concentrations of nerve endings. It has been suggested that acupuncture stimulates large afferent (A beta) nerve fibers that participate in a gate control mechanism in the dorsal horn of the spinal cord, preventing the transmission of pain impulses from afferent A delta and C fibers. Acupuncture also may induce the release of endogenous opioid-like substances such as enkephalins, which decrease the production of substance P in the dorsal horn of the spinal cord, and endorphins, which mediate pain perception via activation of opiate receptors in the brain and spinal cord. Repeated treatments are typically necessary to induce an effect; therefore, the use of acupuncture is mainly restricted to the treatment of chronic pain.

Nursing Care

The stress of hospitalization can contribute to a patient's perception of pain. It is important to provide a comfortable surface that is clean and dry. Limbs with unstable fractures should be immobilized. If frequent blood sampling is anticipated, a central venous catheter should be placed to limit the number of venipunctures. Efforts should be made to allow restful sleep, and noxious handling should be limited. Other sources of discomfort, such as nausea and dyspnea, should be addressed. Additional factors that may ease the patient's anxiety include family visits, hiding boxes, familiar objects from home, and familiar or appealing food.

Suggested Reading

Mathews KA. Norsteroidal anti-inflammatory analgesics in pain management in dogs and cats. Can Vet J 37:539–545, 1996.

Quandt JE, Rawlings CR. Reducing postoperative pain for dogs: Local anesthetic and analgesic techniques. Compendium 18:101–111, 1996.

Short CE, Poznak AV. Animal pain. New York: Churchill Livingstone, 1992.

Mechanical Ventilation

Armelle DeLaforcade and Elizabeth Rozanski

A Types of Ventilation

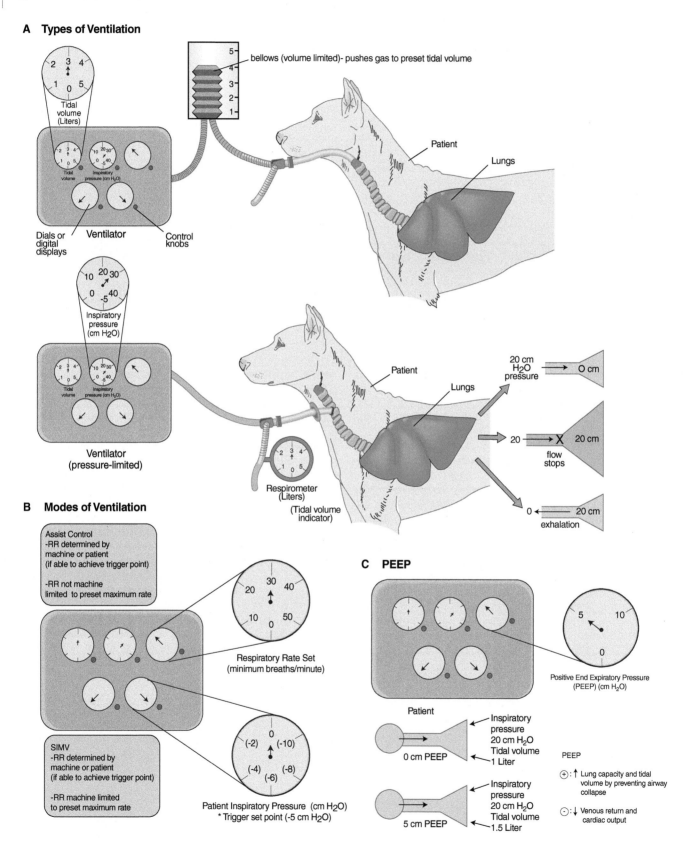

bellows (volume limited)- pushes gas to preset tidal volume

Tidal volume (Liters)

Patient

Lungs

Dials or digital displays

Ventilator

Control knobs

Inspiratory pressure (cm H_2O)

Patient

Lungs

20 cm H_2O pressure → 0 cm

20 → X → 20 cm flow stops

0 ← 20 cm exhalation

Ventilator (pressure-limited)

Respirometer (Liters) (Tidal volume indicator)

B Modes of Ventilation

Assist Control
-RR determined by machine or patient (if able to achieve trigger point)

-RR not machine limited to preset maximum rate

Respiratory Rate Set (minimum breaths/minute)

SIMV
-RR determined by machine or patient (if able to achieve trigger point)

-RR machine limited to preset maximum rate

Patient Inspiratory Pressure (cm H_2O)
* Trigger set point (-5 cm H_2O)

C PEEP

Positive End Expiratory Pressure (PEEP) (cm H_2O)

Patient

Inspiratory pressure 20 cm H_2O Tidal volume 1 Liter

0 cm PEEP

Inspiratory pressure 20 cm H_2O Tidal volume 1.5 Liter

5 cm PEEP

PEEP

⊕ : ↑ Lung capacity and tidal volume by preventing airway collapse

⊖ : ↓ Venous return and cardiac output

Mechanical ventilation is used in the emergency setting in response to a respiratory crisis. In general, mechanical ventilation is indicated when the patient is unable to maintain either a PaO_2 of greater than 50 mmHg despite supplemental oxygen or a PCO_2 of less than 50 mmHg despite reversal of respiratory depressant drugs or thoracocentesis if indicated. This is referred to as the "50/50 rule". Other indications for mechanical ventilation include clinical deterioration of respiratory status to the point of imminent respiratory failure, or respiratory support post cardiopulmonary arrest.

Methods for artificial ventilation range from a simple Ambu-bag attached to an endotracheal tube to a computerized ventilator designed for long-term respiratory support. This chapter will focus on the use of the computerized ventilator since it provides better control over ventilatory variables including oxygen level, humidity, tidal volume, and inspiratory pressure, than a manually operated ventilator.

Types of Ventilation

In general, there are two types of ventilation used in veterinary medicine (**Part A**). Volume limited ventilation is used to deliver a set volume of air to the patient regardless of the pressure required to do so. Pressure alarms are set to detect sudden increases in airway pressures and usually indicate an obstruction. Pressure limited ventilation means that the ventilator will deliver air to a preset inspiratory pressure regardless of the volume that is given. Since there is a tendency for decreased lung compliance with this type of ventilation, $PaCO_2$ and tidal volume are closely monitored (using blood gas measurements and spirometry, respectively). This type of ventilation may be more desirable in very small animals (<10 pounds).

In addition to these two types of ventilation, several modes of mechanical ventilation are available (**Part B**). The Assist/Control mode allows the ventilator to deliver a set number of breaths per minute. These breaths are delivered if the patient is not breathing (at the preset rate), or if the patient generates negative inspiratory pressure. If the patient is breathing rapidly or panting, each shallow breath is converted to a full breath and hyperventilation may result. If this occurs, Synchronous Intermittent Mandatory Ventilation (SIMV) may be a better choice. In this mode the ventilator will also deliver a set number of breaths per minute. The breath may be initiated by negative inspiratory pressure but if the patient breathes faster than the set rate, the machine will not deliver additional breaths. This mode is useful in the weaning process as the number of breaths delivered by the ventilator can be slowly decreased. Spontaneous ventilation is the third option available. In this mode, the ventilator functions similarly to an anesthesia machine. Although not commonly used in veterinary medicine, this mode of ventilation can be useful if set concentrations of oxygen are to be given or following weaning from ventilatory support.

Drugs Used in Ventilation

Many different drugs and protocols have been used to sedate an animal for mechanical ventilation. In many dogs, pentobarbital (2–16 mg/kg IV q 4–6 hours) has been used successfully. Pentobarbital has the advantage of having a long duration of action and relatively low cost. Disadvantages include long recovery phase and lack of reversal agents. Other commonly used drugs include a combination of oxymorphone (0.05–0.1 mg/kg IV prn) and diazepam (0.25–0.5 mg/kg IV prn). Opiates are cardiovascularly sparing but require frequent dosing and are expensive. Other protocols include continuous rate infusions of fentanyl or propofol (to effect). Occasionally neuromuscular blockers such as atracarium (0.2 mg/kg IV) are used to facilitate mechanical ventilation in conjunction with analgesic agents.

Types of Airways

The clinician managing a patient on the ventilator also has the choice of type of airway. The two main choices are oral intubation and tracheostomy tube. The advantages of oral intubation include speed, familiarity and decreased tissue trauma. The primary disadvantages include the need for absolute sedation and immobility. The tracheostomy tube requires less sedation and leaves the potential for oral intake of food and water. Disadvantages of the tracheostomy tube include a surgical procedure on a likely immunocompromised patient and a need for more careful monitoring than in an anesthetised patient (due to potential tube occlusions or dislodgement). In general, if a patient is likely to be ventilated for more than 36–48 hours, it is reasonable to consider a tracheostomy.

Positive end expiratory pressure (PEEP) is an option for patients that are hypoxemic despite a high concentration of inspired oxygen and a normal to low $PaCO_2$ PEEP can improve oxygenation by preventing complete expiration (**Part C**). This results in an increased functional residual capacity, prevents early closure of small airways, and increases alveolar size and perfusion. Important undesirable side effects of PEEP include decrease of venous return to the heart and decreased cardiac output.

Risks

Mechanical ventilation is not risk free. The two primary problems encountered with mechanical ventilation include barotrauma and infection. Barotrauma results from excessive positive pressure developing in certain areas of the lung resulting in rupture and subsequent pneumothorax (or pneumomediastinum) (see Chapter 42). One of the most common causes of desaturation in a previously stable ventilator patient is the development of a significant pneumothorax. A pneumothorax should be anticipated in an animal with significant lung disease, and clients and staff should be counseled not to consider it a major setback.

Infection is another common problem in the ventilated patient. Infections often spread to the lungs from the contamination of the upper airway and oropharynx since the normal defense mechanisms of the upper airway are inhibited. Ventilator patients are often immunosuppressed which also increases their risk of infection. In addition to maintaining aseptic technique, cultures of the airway should be performed every 24–48 hours. Antimicrobial therapy should be used according to culture results and clinical signs. Other potential risks include decreased venous return, oxygen toxicity, upper airway damage and musculoskeletal problems associated with prolonged recumbency.

Prognosis for ventilated animals depends of the underlying disease. Young animals with reversible disease may have a fair prognosis as opposed to older animals with recurrent severe airway diseases that are approaching respiratory failure. In general a survival rate of 30–40% with a good quality of life should be the goal.

General initial settings:
   FiO2: 1.0 (100%) initially, then decrease as soon as possible
   Rate: usually 15–25 breaths per minute initially
   Inspiratory time: I:E ratio should be > 1:1 (inspiration should always be shorter than expiration). Inspiratory time usually starts 0.8–1.5 then maintain appropriate ratio
   Tidal volume: 10 ml/kg Adjust flow rate to appropriate tidal volume

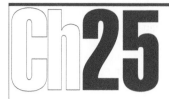

Neuroendocrine Response to and Initial Management of Traumatic Injury

Lisa L. Powell

A

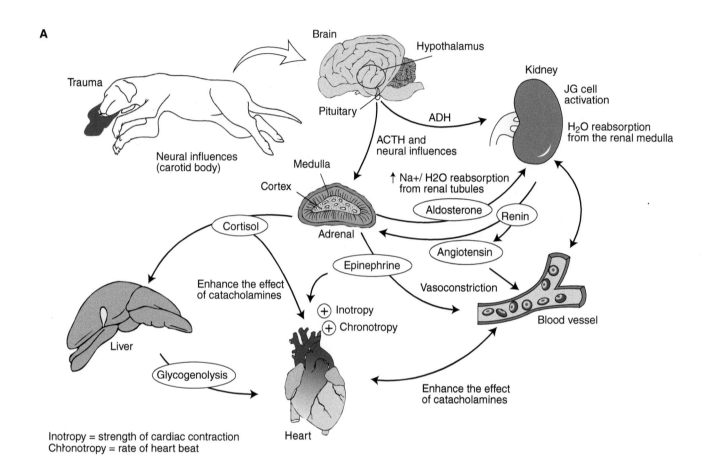

Inotropy = strength of cardiac contraction
Chronotropy = rate of heart beat

B

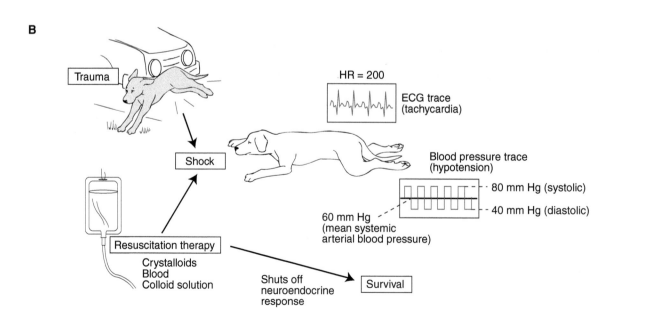

Traumatic injury often results in hypovolemic shock and is responsible for significant morbidity and mortality in canine and feline patients. Naturally occurring compensatory mechanisms stimulated by major trauma exist in an attempt to restore effective circulating volume and maintain vital organ perfusion. Initial compensation includes stimulation of stretch receptors in the carotid arteries and aortic arch, shunting of interstitial fluid into the intravascular space, and the release of hormones and other mediators into the bloodstream. Intravascular fluid loss (i.e., from hemorrhage or maldistribution of blood) results in a decrease in arterial blood pressure, which is detected by baroreceptors in the carotid bodies and aortic arch. In turn, the sympathetic nervous system is activated, causing release of epinephrine and norepinephrine from the adrenal medulla (**Part A**). Adrenocorticotropic hormone (ACTH) is released from the hypothalamus and acts on the adrenal cortex to produce cortisol. The hypothalamus also secretes antidiuretic hormone (ADH) into the circulation. The renin-angiotensin-aldosterone (RAA) system is activated and contributes to restoration of effective intravascular volume.

Compensatory Physiological Responses to Trauma

A release of catecholamines causes an elevation in heart rate and myocardial contractility in an attempt to increase cardiac output. Peripheral vasoconstriction and redistribution of blood to vital organ beds, including the heart, brain, and lungs, occur in response to activation of the sympathetic nervous system. Norepinephrine is a positive inotrope and causes arterial vasoconstriction. Epinephrine promotes hepatic glycogenolysis, lipolysis, and the release of fatty acids and can be used as energy substrates in a shock state.

ACTH is released from the pituitary gland and acts on the adrenal cortex to begin synthesis and release of glucocorticoids, primarily cortisol. Cortisol plays a major role in facilitating adaptation to trauma. Catecholamines and other hormones are able to exert their cardiovascular effects, owing to the permissive action of cortisol. Elevated cortisol levels also cause a rise in plasma osmolality by promoting hyperglycemia, which in turn causes water to be drawn into the interstitial space. The increase in interstitial pressure enhances protein transfer into the vascular system through lymph and venous systems, and helps to restore normal plasma protein levels. Glucocorticoids also inhibit the release of arachidonic acid from cell membranes through inhibition of the enzyme phospholipase A_2. The products of arachidonic acid, including prostaglandins, prostacyclin, leukotrienes, and thromboxane A_2, are inhibited, and their potentially harmful effects (i.e., development of the systemic inflammatory response system) are not achieved. Plasma cortisol levels rise between 2 and 6 hours after a traumatic event. Plasma cortisol levels peak at 24 hours, and may remain elevated for 48–72 hours after the initial traumatic event.

ADH is released into the circulation in response to hypovolemia, hyperosmolality of the blood, water depletion, and hemorrhage. ADH inhibits water diuresis by causing active water resorption in the renal collecting tubules in an attempt to restore normal circulating fluid volume. Thus, urine production is decreased in posttraumatic animals.

The RAA system also is activated following a hypovolemic event. Baroreceptors and sodium-sensitive chemoreceptors are activated in response to hypovolemia and hyperosmolality of the blood and act on the juxtaglomerular cells in the kidney to produce renin. Renin is an enzyme that reacts with angiotensinogen, a plasma-2-globulin, to form angiotensin I. A peptidase, angiotensin-converting enzyme, converts angiotensin I to angiotensin II in the lungs. Angiotensin II stimulates the secretion of aldosterone from the adrenal cortex. Angiotensin II is also a potent vasoconstrictor. Aldosterone promotes the renal retention of sodium, and therefore water, and thus causes an increase in intravascular volume.

Intervention

The mainstay of treatment for animals following a traumatic event and presenting in hypovolemic shock is IV fluid therapy (**Part B**). Animals in hypovolemic shock are tachycardic and tachypneic, have weak arterial pulse quality, have pale mucous membranes, are hypothermic in response to decreased perfusion, and may be mentally dull due to cerebral hypoperfusion and hypoxia. Treatment can be tailored according to the specific injuries and the amount of blood loss. Colloid support and hypertonic saline solution often are administered in animals that are severely hypovolemic or have significant blood protein losses. Blood transfusions should be considered in patients with significant blood loss and, as a general rule of thumb, have a packed cell volume (PCV) <25%–30%. Animals with pulmonary injuries may be more sensitive to excessive fluid administration; however, fluids should not be restricted in these patients, and fluids sufficient to support blood pressure, central venous pressure, and adequate urine output should be administered. The treatment of hypovolemic shock with glucocorticoids has long been a debatable issue. No clinical studies have shown a benefit to the use of glucocorticoids in posttraumatic, hypovolemic animals or humans. Glucocorticoid administration clearly should be administered in situations in which a deficiency of cortisol exists, such as in an animal with a history of hypoadrenocorticism (Addison's disease) or chronic steroid administration (iatrogenic hypoadrenocorticism).

Conclusion

Many compensatory mechanisms are activated following a traumatic event. Trauma that results in hypovolemic shock causes decreased perfusion to tissues, with subsequent tissue and cellular hypoxia. The primary goal of these compensatory mechanisms is to restore circulating blood volume and allow for normal tissue perfusion and oxygenation. When these compensatory mechanisms are overwhelmed or are inadequate to support normal blood pressure and tissue perfusion, medical intervention becomes necessary. Prolonged shock causes death secondary to hypoxia to vital organs, including the heart, lungs, and brain. The recognition and appropriate treatment of hypovolemic shock following a traumatic event is imperative to avoid hypoxic damage to tissues and possibly death of the patient. A clear understanding of the neuroendocrine response to trauma assists the veterinary practitioner's approach to the posttraumatic patient.

Ch26 Stressed Starvation and Nutritional Assessment

Andrea Gilbert and Robert J. Murtaugh

A

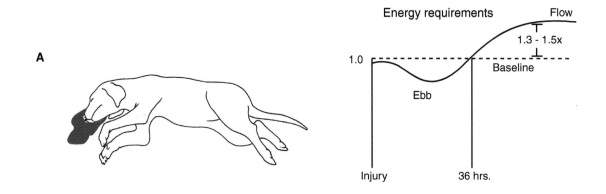

Energy requirements

1.0

Ebb

Injury

36 hrs.

Flow

1.3 - 1.5x

Baseline

B Hypermetabolism

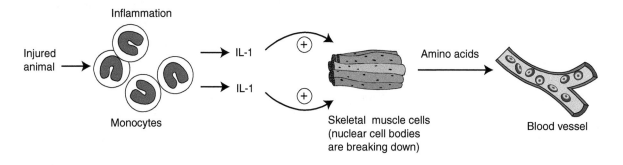

Inflammation

Injured animal

IL-1

IL-1

+

+

Monocytes

Amino acids

Skeletal muscle cells
(nuclear cell bodies
are breaking down)

Blood vessel

C

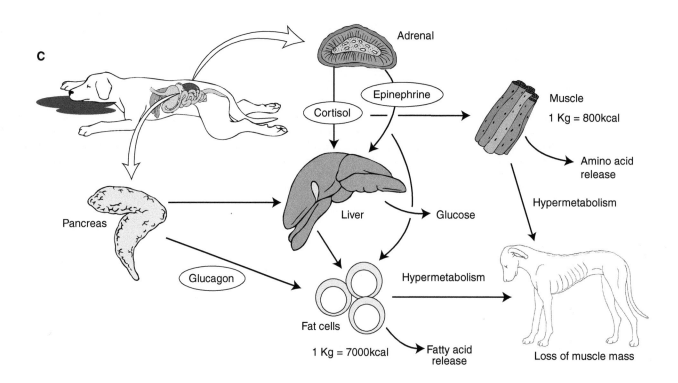

Adrenal

Epinephrine

Cortisol

Muscle
1 Kg = 800kcal

Amino acid
release

Hypermetabolism

Liver

Glucose

Pancreas

Glucagon

Fat cells

1 Kg = 7000kcal

Fatty acid
release

Hypermetabolism

Loss of muscle mass

Injury and illness result in metabolic alterations. These alterations are very different from the endocrine and metabolic events of uncomplicated starvation. Sick or injured animals are hypermetabolic, while with uncomplicated starvation, metabolic rate decreases. A simple explanation of the metabolic alterations that occur after injury is the ebb and flow theory (**Part A**). The ebb phase lasts 24–36 hours after the injury and is characterized by decreased oxygen consumption, lowered body metabolism, and vasoconstriction. The flow phase follows the ebb phase and is characterized by increased metabolic rate, increased body temperature, and accelerated nitrogen loss. During the ebb phase, the major concerns are stabilization of pulmonary and cardiovascular functions. During the flow phase, metabolic and nutritional support should be the primary therapeutic concerns.

Pathophysiology of Hypermetabolism

A number of metabolic changes occur during illness or injury, and these changes act together to produce the hypermetabolic state (**Part B**). Cytokines play a role in the metabolic changes seen during critical illness. Tumor necrosis factor (TNF) and interleukin (IL)-1 are 2 cytokines that are important during sepsis and injury. IL-1 is synthesized by macrophages and monocytes. This cytokine acts on muscle tissue to increase proteolysis. These actions are mediated by prostaglandin E_2. TNF is released by stimulated macrophages and has many physiological effects that are similar to those of IL-1. It is a major mediator of the effects of endotoxin.

Three hormones—glucagon, catecholamines, and cortisol—mediate much of the metabolic change that occurs following injury or onset of illness (**Part C**). These hormones are called *counter regulatory hormones,* opposing the action on insulin. Insulin is the predominant hormone in the normal physiological state. The release of these hormones and involved cytokines is stimulated by local tissue injury and inflammation or by disturbances in homeostasis such as hypovolemia, hypoglycemia, or acidosis.

Glucocorticoids, catecholamines, and glucagon contribute to the insulin resistance observed in stressed metabolic states. Gluconeogenesis is not suppressed despite high blood glucose and insulin concentrations, hepatic glucose production continues, and blood glucagon levels remain elevated (see **Part C**). These counterregulatory hormones also promote lipolysis and mobilization of amino acids from muscle. These processes are not responsive to the administration of exogenous glucose.

Fat oxidation is an important source of energy in hypermetabolic patients. Tissues in the body use fatty acids in response to the influence of the counterregulatory hormones. The persistently high level of glucose production and insulin concentration limits ketogenesis in these patients. The brain in patients with hypermetabolism must rely on glucose for energy, in comparison to the brain of a fasted, but unstressed, animal that would rely on ketones for energy. This CNS need for glucose largely determines the amount of muscle protein catabolism required to fuel ongoing gluconeogenesis.

Clinically, septic and critically injured patients exhibit a wasting syndrome that will occur despite adequate calorie intake. This phenomenon occurs without necessarily observing an elevation of metabolic rate, but rather as a metabolic reaction to injury driven by the release of cytokines and the counterregulatory hormones that stimulate the use of muscle for fuel. One kilogram of muscle provides 800 kcal while 1 kg of fat provides 7,000 kcal. Muscle catabolism for use in energy production can cause dramatic wasting without the presence of an increased metabolic rate. This muscle proteolysis is needed to provide specific nutrients that cannot be derived from fat. In addition to the glucose required by the brain, the liver and the hematopoietic tissues require amino acids to synthesize acute-phase proteins and increase production of white blood cells. Nitrogen wasting occurs as glucocorticoids, catecholamines, and glucagon cause nitrogen loss by the kidney that is a reflection of the persistent amino acid mobilization from skeletal muscle.

Nutritional Assessment

In an effort to limit the detrimental effects of the metabolic response to energy and nutrient requirements in patients with critical illness, nutritional assessment and intervention should be practiced in all these patients. A number of different parameters can be used to assess the baseline nutritional status and ongoing nutritional support needs of critically ill animals. Body weight is an easily monitored parameter indicating a patient's basal nutritional state. Nutritional support should be considered if the animal has recently lost >10% of its optimal body weight. Even if an animal is initially obese, weight loss (muscle catabolism) is not desirable during critical illness. Physical examination findings that point to preexistent or ongoing nutritional deficiencies include dry, flaky skin; lusterless, thin coat of hair; poor wound healing; and pressure sores. Laboratory parameters such as albumin level, lymphocyte count, packed cell volume, and BUN concentration can be a reflection of nutritional status.

Anorexia for >3 days represents an indication for nutritional intervention in a hospitalized patient without historical weight loss or persistent nutritional deficiency. Patients that are anticipated to be unable to or unwilling to eat on their own within 3 days of diagnosis or intervention (e.g., extensive GI resection, pancreatitis, head injury) are candidates for nutritional support. Additionally, patients whose condition results in nutrient loss (chylothorax, open abdomen, large draining wounds) require careful ongoing evaluation and support of nutritional status.

Conclusion

Critically ill animals require the same consideration for their nutritional needs as that necessary for resuscitative management of hemodynamic, respiratory, and other organ system dysfunction. The morbidity and mortality associated with critical illness can be influenced directly through addressing the nutritional support requirements of these patients.

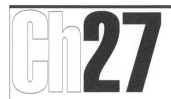

Ch27 Feeding the Critically Ill Patient

Andrea Gilbert and Robert J. Murtaugh

Feeding the Critically Ill Patient

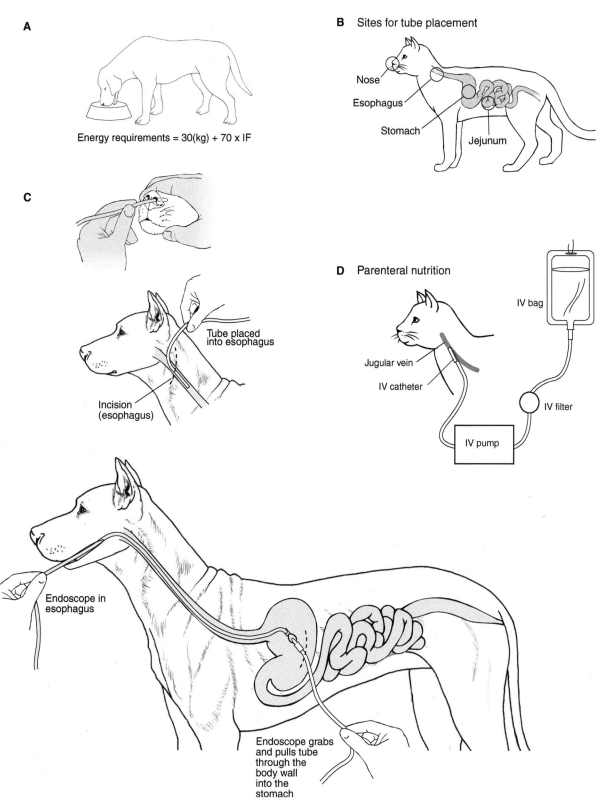

A

Energy requirements = 30(kg) + 70 x IF

B Sites for tube placement

Nose
Esophagus
Stomach
Jejunum

C

Tube placed into esophagus

Incision (esophagus)

D Parenteral nutrition

IV bag
Jugular vein
IV catheter
IV filter
IV pump

Endoscope in esophagus

Endoscope grabs and pulls tube through the body wall into the stomach

When the clinician has decided to use nutritional support, the specifics need to be addressed. The route for nutritional support administration needs to be decided. A basic guideline is to use the enteral route whenever possible. Parenteral nutrition should be used when the GI tract is not functioning or when it is not possible to obtain a route to administer enteral nutrition.

The value for resting energy requirements (RERs) needs to be calculated. Two formulas are used to calculate RER: $70 \times$ Weight (in kg)$^{0.75}$ = kcal/day; and $30 \times$ Weight (in kg) + 70 (**Part A**).

Once RER has been calculated, the illness energy requirement (IER) is calculated by multiplying an illness factor (IF) by the RER: IER = RER $\times$ IF. The IF takes into account the estimated increased energy needs during illness; for most patients the IF = 1.1–1.3. The IF should be figured conservatively, with 1.5 being the maximum, reserved for severely septic or burn-injured animals.

Enteral Nutrition

Enteral Feeding Routes

Enteral route choices include force feeding or use of a nasoesophageal (NE) tube, esophagostomy tube, gastrostomy tube, and jejunostomy tube (**Part B**). If the upper GI tract is functional and nutritional support is likely needed for <1 week, an NE tube represents a logical choice.

With the aid of local anesthesia, an NE tube can be placed into the nostrils (**Part C**). A radiograph is helpful to confirm correct placement of the end of the tube in the distal end of the esophagus. A liquid, polymeric enteral diet formulated for use in dogs and cats is recommended for feeding through NE tubes in order to prevent tube clogging. Complications associated with the use of NE tubes include nasal irritation, regurgitation of feedings, and migration of the tube into the airway.

Use of an esophagostomy tube is another option for providing short-term enteral feeding. It is surgically inserted through the cervical esophagus, with the distal end placed into the lower part of the esophagus. This enteral route can be helpful in patients with mandibular or maxillary fractures when they are not able to prehend food. Potential complications include regurgitation, esophageal irritation, gastroesophageal reflux, and pneumonia.

Stomach tubes can be placed by surgical, endoscopic, or blind insertion techniques. Whenever intra-abdominal surgical intervention is indicated in a critically ill animal with nutritional support needs, the clinician should consider placement of a gastrostomy tube. These feeding tubes can be maintained in place and utilized for extended periods of time. It is important to place large-bore tubes (18–22F for a cat, 20–30F for a dog) as smaller-bore tubes can clog more readily. Major complications of gastrostomy tubes include insertion site infection and peritonitis. These tubes should be left in place for a minimum of 7–10 days prior to consideration for removal. This practice will ensure a good seal to form between the stomach and the body wall, minimizing the chance of postextraction peritonitis.

Jejunostomy tubes also are placed surgically and are indicated if the upper GI tract is nonfunctional. These tubes require more intensive care to maintain than is usually necessary with other enteral feeding tubes. A liquid diet must be used with this enteral route, and the diet is best administered by continuous infusion rather than by bolus feeding.

Enteral Feeding Practices

Following placement of an enteral feeding tube, the next steps are to select an enteral diet, establish the kilocalories per milliliter the diet contains, and then calculate the daily amount of the diet the patient requires to meet the IER. When enteral feedings are initiated, one-third of the calculated IER is administered on day 1. The amount is increased to two-thirds of IER on day 2 and up to full requirements on day 3. These enteral formulations should be warmed and given slowly. Enteral feeding tubes should be flushed with a small amount (5 mL) of warm water before and after feeding. Before feeding, stomach tubes should be aspirated, and if large residual volumes (greater than half the feeding volume) are in the stomach, the current feeding should be withheld and then subsequent feedings should be smaller and at more frequent intervals. If the animal coughs or vomits, feeding should be temporarily suspended. The placement of NE or esophagostomy tubes should be checked carefully in these circumstances. In animals that have been anorexic for an extended period of time, it is important to estimate nutritional requirements conservatively and slowly increase feedings to calculated requirements over 1–2 weeks, to avoid the refeeding syndrome.

Parenteral Nutrition

With parenteral nutrition, a mixture of lipid, amino acid, and dextrose solutions compounded under sterile conditions supplies the calculated energy needs of the patient. Parenteral nutrition can be total (TPN) or partial (PPN). TPN supplies the complete energy requirements of the animal.

TPN

TPN should be initiated gradually: one-third of calculated requirements the first day, two-thirds the second day, and full requirements the third day. TPN must be administered through a dedicated central venous line (see **Part D**) to maintain aseptic administration and minimize thrombophlebitis due to the hyperosmolar character of TPN solutions. Parenteral nutrition formulations provide a good medium for bacterial growth; therefore, a dedicated line should be used and the connections should be maintained aseptically.

PPN

PPN supplies about half of a patient's energy requirement. It is best for short-term nutritional support or to supplement enteral alimentation and limited, but inadequate, oral intake by the critically ill patient. A central venous line is not necessary for PPN administration as the solutions are not hyperosmolar, but the use of a dedicated line and aseptic technique in handling the administration of PPN is essential.

Special Considerations

Vitamin and mineral requirements need to be met by administration of nutritional support to critically ill animals receiving TPN or PPN. The recommendation is to administer 0.5 mg of vitamin K/kg subcutaneously on the day TPN or PPN is initiated and then to administer once-weekly doses. B complex vitamins and trace minerals should be administered daily to these patients as well. Cats have unique dietary requirements that include taurine, arachidonic acid, and vitamin A.

During the administration of parenteral nutrition, the GI tract is not being exposed to intraluminal dietary fiber or glutamine, an essential nutrient necessary for intestinal cell growth and replication. Therefore, intestinal mucosal atrophy often accompanies parenteral feeding. The intestinal mucosa is a protective barrier to intraluminal bacteria and toxins in normal, healthy animals. Even when an animal is receiving parenteral nutrition, consideration should be given to administering a small amount of a glutamine-enriched or short-chain-fatty-acid–enriched solution through an NE tube to promote intestinal health and minimize bacterial translocation.

Conclusion

The provision of energy and nutrients to critically ill animals requires consideration of enteral and parenteral nutrition approaches. The patient's IER and other nutritional considerations can be met through administration by either route or by a combination of enteral and parenteral nutrition. Careful planning, administration, and monitoring of nutritional support procedures are required to minimize complications and ensure successful treatment.

Ch28 CCPR: Airway/Breathing/Circulation

Jeffrey Proulx

CCPR Crash Cart and Equipment

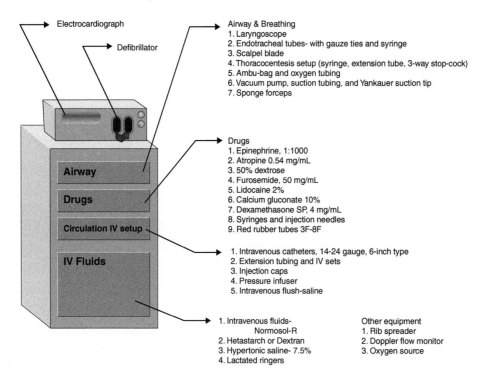

Electrocardiograph

Defibrillator

Airway & Breathing
1. Laryngoscope
2. Endotracheal tubes- with gauze ties and syringe
3. Scalpel blade
4. Thoracocentesis setup (syringe, extension tube, 3-way stop-cock)
5. Ambu-bag and oxygen tubing
6. Vacuum pump, suction tubing, and Yankauer suction tip
7. Sponge forceps

Airway

Drugs

Circulation IV setup

IV Fluids

Drugs
1. Epinephrine, 1:1000
2. Atropine 0.54 mg/mL
3. 50% dextrose
4. Furosemide, 50 mg/mL
5. Lidocaine 2%
6. Calcium gluconate 10%
7. Dexamethasone SP, 4 mg/mL
8. Syringes and injection needles
9. Red rubber tubes 3F-8F

1. Intravenous catheters, 14-24 gauge, 6-inch type
2. Extension tubing and IV sets
3. Injection caps
4. Pressure infuser
5. Intravenous flush-saline

1. Intravenous fluids-
   Normosol-R
2. Hetastarch or Dextran
3. Hypertonic saline- 7.5%
4. Lactated ringers

Other equipment
1. Rib spreader
2. Doppler flow monitor
3. Oxygen source

The Equipment Required to Maintain Airway/Breathing
Endotracheal tubes with preplaced gauze tie and syringe for cuff inflation
Laryngoscope with small and large blades
Vacuum pump with suction apparatus/tubing and Yankauer suction tip
Ambu bag with oxygen tubing and oxygen source
Tracheostomy setup (scalpel blade and suture material)
Thoracocentesis setup (3-way stop-cock, IV extension tubing, 60-cc syringe, and injection needle)
Sponge forceps for foreign body removal
Thoracostomy tubes: sizes 16F-36F

The Equipment Required to Maintain Circulation
IV Catheters (1-2 inch over-the-needle type): sizes 14-25 gauge
IV fluids: crystalloid (0.9 NaCl, Normosol, or Plasmalyte) and hypertonic saline 7.5%
IV Fluids: colloids (dextran-70 or 6% hetastarch)
IV sets, extension tubing, injection caps, 1-inch white tape
Pressure bag or rapid infuser
IV cutdown setup (scalpel and suture material)
Open-chest CCPR setup (rib retractors, scalpel blade, Mayo scissors, vascular clamp)
ECG, Doppler flow monitor/transducer
Defibrillator

The Drug Dosage Chart

		Indications
Epinephrine	0.02-0.2mg/kg	Ventricular fibrillation, asystole, EMD
Atropine	0.04 mg/kg	Bradyarrhythmias, ventricular asystole
Dextrose 50%	1 mL/kg	Hypoglycemia
Calcium gluconate 10%	1 mL/kg	Hyperkalemia, hypermagnesemia; calcium channel blocker overdose; hypocalcemia
Sodium bicarbonate	1 mEq/kg	CCPR > 5 minutes
Furosemide	2-6 mg/kg	Cardiogenic pulmonary edema
Lidocaine	2-8 mg/kg	Post resuscitation ventricular tachyarrhythmia (not ventricular fibrillation)
Defibrillation	2-10 J/kg	External shock for ventricular fibrillation

Cardiopulmonary arrest (CPA) has many causes that can include trauma, drugs and anesthetics, metabolic disturbances, neurological disorders, and other primary cardiorespiratory disorders. Cardiac arrest can occur secondary to a primary respiratory arrest or result from dysrhythmia. With cessation of blood flow, tissue hypoxia results in the depletion of intracellular energy stores and ATP within 4–5 minutes. With continued hypoxia, intracellular acidosis, increases in intracellular calcium, and irreversible cellular damage occur. Resuscitative efforts are aimed at supporting cerebral and myocardial oxygenation to maintain neurological integrity and obtain a spontaneous return of circulatory function.

Patient Considerations

Several factors should be considered before performing cardiopulmonary resuscitation. These include the age of the patient, the time elapsed since the CPA, the primary cause of the arrest (if known), reversibility of the disease, and the long-term prognosis. Additionally, it is important to consider the client's wishes, as well as staff and hospital capabilities to perform and care for a patient that has had a CPA.

Approach

Readiness
Successful resuscitation necessitates appropriate equipment and qualified personnel. This includes a well-organized cerebral-cardiopulmonary resuscitation (CCPR) station and crash cart (**Figure**) to perform basic and advanced resuscitation. The hospital staff must be trained in CCPR techniques and procedures and be able to perform efficiently as a team.

Recognition
Patients at risk for CPA should be identified either by phone or physical triage (for patients coming or presenting to the hospital), or based on disease and clinical condition (for patients already being treated in the hospital). Respiratory arrest or agonal breathing patterns, cyanosis, and lack of auscultable heart beat or palpable pulse are some clear indications to begin resuscitative efforts.

Airway and Breathing
The first step in approaching a CPA patient is to secure the airway. This includes an airway exam with laryngoscope. If an upper-airway obstruction is identified, removal of the foreign body or slash tracheostomy may be necessary. Without obstructive pathology, the patient should be intubated quickly and manual ventilation begun at 20–30 bpm with an AMBU bag attached to oxygen at a high flow rate, or 100% oxygen given through a nonrebreathing anesthetic or ventilator circuit. Examination of chest excursion and bilateral chest auscultation should be performed to ensure adequate ventilation and proper endotracheal (ET) tube placement. High resistance to ventilation should prompt evaluation for pleural space disease (e.g., pneumothorax) or conditions with lowered lung compliance (e.g., pulmonary edema). Thoracocentesis may distinguish between the 2 disorders; emergency thoracotomy or chest tube placement may be necessary

to allow adequate ventilation. Proper suction equipment must be available if it is necessary to remove fluid and debris at the time of intubation, or if pulmonary edema fluid discharges through the ET tube. Postural drainage (lifting the body higher than the head and neck) may also help in removing fluid in patients with copious amounts of pulmonary edema.

Circulation
The necessity of chest compression needs to be assessed by examination of ECG and clinical evaluation of adequate perfusion (evidence of auscultable heart beat and palpable pulses). Circulatory support should be initiated only after the airway is secured and adequate ventilatory support is instituted. Chest compression is begun at approximately 80–100 compressions/min in larger patients (>10 kg) or 120 compressions/min in patients <10 kg. Although controversial, the cardiac pump mechanism probably is more important in generating blood flow in patients <10 kg; therefore, compressions should be performed with the patient in lateral recumbency, and directly over the heart. Larger patients should have compressions performed at the widest aspect of the chest, potentially giving the maximal amount of increased intrathoracic pressure. Compressions with the patient in dorsal recumbency may accomplish this task, as long as the patient can be stabilized adequately in this position. The optimal compression-relaxation proportion (duty cycle) is typically 50%/50%. The effectiveness of thoracic compressions should be evaluated intermittently and the technique adjusted to maximize perfusion. Simple measures to evaluate circulation include pulse detection, detection of orbital vessel blood flow by Doppler ultrasound transducer, end-tidal carbon dioxide measurement (higher value = more effective lung perfusion), and intermittent evaluation of ECG for rhythm. Interposed abdominal compressions may augment central venous return.

Open-chest CCPR should be performed in larger patients when closed-chest compression is ineffective (within 5 minutes) and immediately in patients suffering from thoracic wall injury, intrathoracic tension phenomena (pneumothorax, pneumomediastinum), or pericardial disease. Open-chest CCPR allows for more effective perfusion by performing direct cardiac massage. No patient preparation is performed; an incision is made along the right fifth intercostal space through the skin, subcutaneous tissue, and intercostal musculature down to the parietal pleura. Ventilation is discontinued while penetrating the pleural space with a blunt object such as scissors or a hemostat. The incision is extended dorsally and ventrally to allow a large opening, but care must be taken not to sever the ventral intrathoracic artery, which runs along the lateral aspect of the sternum. The pericardium is incised at the diaphragmatic border and is reflected toward the base of the heart. Additionally the aorta can be cross-clamped to increase aortic pressure, allowing for greater coronary and cerebral perfusion. This is accomplished by reflecting the dorsal aspect of the caudal lung lobe ventrally, and using a vascular clamp or hemostat to grasp a red rubber tube that encircles the aorta. Direct cardiac massage is performed while being careful to prevent rotation of the heart from its normal position, to prevent tearing or kinking of the larger blood vessels.

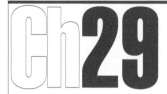

CCPR: Fluids/Drugs/Defibrillation

Jeffrey Proulx

CCPR Crash Cart and Equipment

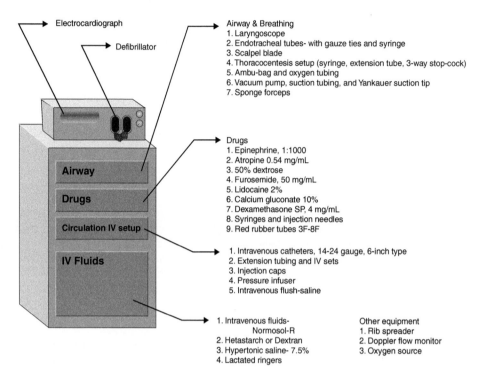

Electrocardiograph

Defibrillator

Airway & Breathing
1. Laryngoscope
2. Endotracheal tubes- with gauze ties and syringe
3. Scalpel blade
4. Thoracocentesis setup (syringe, extension tube, 3-way stop-cock)
5. Ambu-bag and oxygen tubing
6. Vacuum pump, suction tubing, and Yankauer suction tip
7. Sponge forceps

Airway

Drugs

Drugs
1. Epinephrine, 1:1000
2. Atropine 0.54 mg/mL
3. 50% dextrose
4. Furosemide, 50 mg/mL
5. Lidocaine 2%
6. Calcium gluconate 10%
7. Dexamethasone SP, 4 mg/mL
8. Syringes and injection needles
9. Red rubber tubes 3F-8F

Circulation IV setup

1. Intravenous catheters, 14-24 gauge, 6-inch type
2. Extension tubing and IV sets
3. Injection caps
4. Pressure infuser
5. Intravenous flush-saline

IV Fluids

1. Intravenous fluids-
      Normosol-R
2. Hetastarch or Dextran
3. Hypertonic saline- 7.5%
4. Lactated ringers

Other equipment
1. Rib spreader
2. Doppler flow monitor
3. Oxygen source

The Equipment Required to Maintain Airway/Breathing
Endotracheal tubes with preplaced gauze tie and syringe for cuff inflation
Laryngoscope with small and large blades
Vacuum pump with suction apparatus/tubing and Yankauer suction tip
Ambu bag with oxygen tubing and oxygen source
Tracheostomy setup (scalpel blade and suture material)
Thoracocentesis setup (3-way stop-cock, IV extension tubing, 60-cc syringe, and injection needle)
Sponge forceps for foreign body removal
Thoracostomy tubes: sizes 16F-36F

The Equipment Required to Maintain Circulation
IV Catheters (1-2 inch over-the-needle type): sizes 14-25 gauge
IV fluids: crystalloid (0.9 NaCl, Normosol, or Plasmalyte) and hypertonic saline 7.5%
IV Fluids: colloids (dextran-70 or 6% hetastarch)
IV sets, extension tubing, injection caps, 1-inch white tape
Pressure bag or rapid infuser
IV cutdown setup (scalpel and suture material)
Open-chest CCPR setup (rib retractors, scalpel blade, Mayo scissors, vascular clamp)
ECG, Doppler flow monitor/transducer
Defibrillator

The Drug Dosage Chart

		Indications
Epinephrine	0.02-0.2mg/kg	Ventricular fibrillation, asystole, EMD
Atropine	0.04 mg/kg	Bradyarrhythmias, ventricular asystole
Dextrose 50%	1 mL/kg	Hypoglycemia
Calcium gluconate 10%	1 mL/kg	Hyperkalemia, hypermagnesemia; calcium channel blocker overdose; hypocalcemia
Sodium bicarbonate	1 mEq/kg	CCPR > 5 minutes
Furosemide	2-6 mg/kg	Cardiogenic pulmonary edema
Lidocaine	2-8 mg/kg	Post resuscitation ventricular tachyarrhythmia (not ventricular fibrillation)
Defibrillation	2-10 J/kg	External shock for ventricular fibrillation

Cardiopulmonary arrest (CPA) has many causes that can include trauma, drugs and anesthetics, metabolic disturbances, neurological disorders, and other primary cardiorespiratory disorders. Cardiac arrest can occur secondary to a primary respiratory arrest or result from dysrhythmia. With cessation of blood flow, tissue hypoxia results in the depletion of intracellular energy stores and ATP within 4–5 minutes. With continued hypoxia, intracellular acidosis, increases in intracellular calcium, and irreversible cellular damage occur. Resuscitative efforts are aimed at supporting cerebral and myocardial oxygenation to maintain neurological integrity and obtain a spontaneous return of circulatory function.

IV Access and Fluids

IV access should be obtained after basic CCPR measures are started. Central venous access (e.g., jugular catheterization) is preferable to peripheral locations. A venous cutdown should be performed if initial attempts at percutaneous catheterization are unsuccessful. The amount and rate of fluid administration are controversial. During CPA, systemic vasodilation occurs, leading to a condition of relative hypovolemia. In comparison, coronary perfusion depends on a gradient of aortic to right atrial pressure (coronary perfusion = aortic pressure − right atrial pressure). Because IV fluids may increase right atrial filling pressure, and therefore limit coronary perfusion, take care when administering IV fluids. Fluids administered aggressively are generally recommended during initiation of CCPR unless pulmonary or systemic venous congestion is thought to be related to the cause of CPA.

Drugs

Although controversial, high-dose epinephrine (0.2 mg/kg) is probably more effective in CCPR than low-dose epinephrine administration (0.02 mg/kg) (**Figure**). Epinephrine is given every 3–5 minutes IV (preferably in a central vein). Alternatively, the dose may be multiplied by 2–10 and administered into the distal end of the trachea with a syringe and red rubber tube if IV access is not obtained. The main beneficial effect of epinephrine is its $\alpha 1$-agonist action effecting systemic vasoconstriction, ultimately increasing arterial pressure and supporting cerebral and coronary perfusion. Additionally, the β_2 action may dilate coronary and cerebral arterioles, further augmenting blood flow to these areas. Because high-dose epinephrine is associated with a higher incidence of postresuscitation tachyarrhythmia and fibrillation, high-dose epinephrine should only be used in facilities equipped with an electrical defibrillator.

Atropine may be beneficial in patients with CPA caused by high vagal tone, or in patients with bradyarrhythmias, electromechanical dissociation, (EMD) and ventricular asystole during CCPR attempts.

The use of sodium bicarbonate is reserved for patients known to have had a CPA secondary to metabolic acidosis, or patients undergoing prolonged CCPR. The current recommendation is to administer sodium bicarbonate after each 5 minutes of CCPR. Potential complications of therapy include hypercapnia and worsening acidosis if ventilation is not adequate; paradoxical cellular acidosis; hypokalemia; hypernatremia; and shifting of the oxygen dissociation curve to the left.

Dextrose (50%) should be included in the crash cart as many patients have hypoglycemia associated with a CPA. This is especially common in neonates, geriatric patients, and patients with neoplasia and sepsis.

Historically, calcium was recommended as a treatment during CCPR for patients with, electro-mechanical dissociation (EMD) or patients unresponsive to CCPR efforts. With the knowledge that higher concentrations of cellular calcium are cytotoxic, combined with deranged cellular calcium regulation in hypoxic cells, calcium therapy is no longer recommended as a main drug for use in CCPR. IV calcium therapy should be used in CPA patients with associated hyperkalemia, hypocalcemia, calcium channel overdose, or hypermagnesemia.

Lidocaine use is reserved for postresuscitation ventricular tachyarrhythmias. It is no longer recommended for use in ventricular fibrillation, as lidocaine *increases* the defibrillation threshold.

Other drugs commonly kept in a crash cart include bretylium, diltiazem, propanolol, dopamine, dobutamine, furosemide, magnesium chloride, and naloxone.

Defibrillation

Defibrillation is performed in patients who are confirmed to have fibrillation on the ECG. If a patient has a CPA and fibrillation is known to be the cause, immediate defibrillation is the only resuscitative measure that supercedes securing the airway and institution of chest compressions. The "ABC's" must quickly follow if early defibrillation is unsuccessful. Proper defibrillation includes the use of appropriate electrolyte gel and applying firm pressure to ensure good paddle-skin contact. The patient should be countershocked on a nonconducting surface, and the operator needs to wear gloves and ensure that no one has contact with the patient during countershock. The initial shock delivered for external defibrillation should be in the range of 2–10 Joules/kg. Sequential (rapidly applied) shocks of similar intensity may alleviate ventricular fibrillation when initial shock is ineffective. For internal defibrillation, the dosage of energy is 5–10 Joules initially, scaled up to a maximum of 50 Joules if needed.

Prolonged Support

Patients that regain spontaneous heart rhythm need to have further care to support normal organ function. Initial efforts should be directed at supporting normal body physiology in regards to protecting the cerebral tissue, correcting postresuscitation electrolyte and acid-base disturbances, maintaining systemic hemodynamics, and supporting pulmonary function through controlled mechanical ventilation if necessary. The underlying cause of the CPA should be identified and the primary disease treated accordingly.

Ch30 Shock I: Pathophysiology

James Ross, Robert J. Murtaugh, and Kari Moore

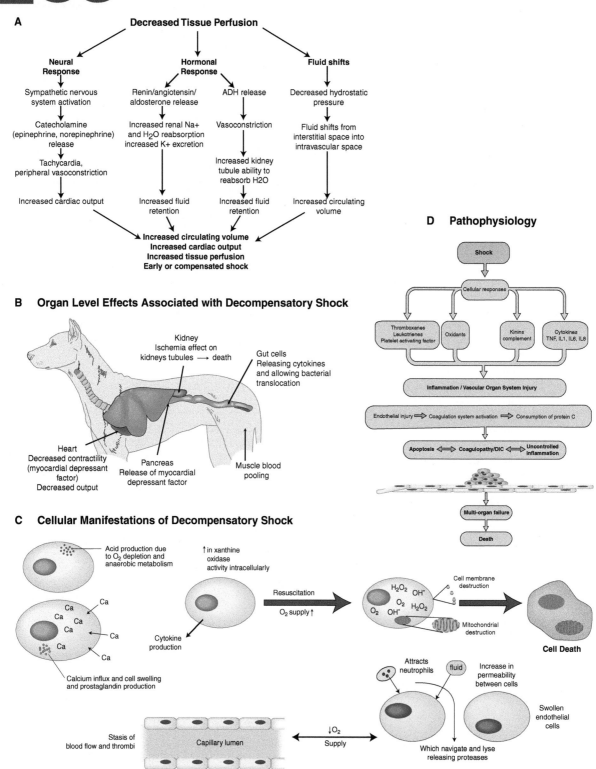

A

Decreased Tissue Perfusion

Neural Response → Sympathetic nervous system activation → Catecholamine (epinephrine, norepinephrine) release → Tachycardia, peripheral vasoconstriction → Increased cardiac output

Hormonal Response → Renin/angiotensin/ aldosterone release → Increased renal Na+ and H_2O reabsorption increased K+ excretion → Increased fluid retention

ADH release → Vasoconstriction → Increased kidney tubule ability to reabsorb H2O → Increased fluid retention

Fluid shifts → Decreased hydrostatic pressure → Fluid shifts from interstitial space into intravascular space → Increased circulating volume

Increased circulating volume
Increased cardiac output
Increased tissue perfusion
Early or compensated shock

B   Organ Level Effects Associated with Decompensatory Shock

Kidney
Ischemia effect on kidneys tubules → death

Gut cells
Releasing cytokines and allowing bacterial translocation

Heart
Decreased contractility (myocardial depressant factor)
Decreased output

Pancreas
Release of myocardial depressant factor

Muscle blood pooling

C   Cellular Manifestations of Decompensatory Shock

Acid production due to O_2 depletion and anaerobic metabolism

↑ in xanthine oxidase activity intracellularly

Ca Ca Ca Ca Ca Ca

Resuscitation
O_2 supply ↑

H_2O_2 OH⁻ O_2 H_2O_2 O_2 OH⁻

Cell membrane destruction

Mitochondrial destruction

Cell Death

Cytokine production

Calcium influx and cell swelling and prostaglandin production

Attracts neutrophils

fluid

Increase in permeability between cells

Swollen endothelial cells

Stasis of blood flow and thrombi

Capillary lumen

↓O_2 Supply

Which navigate and lyse releasing proteases

D   Pathophysiology

Shock → Cellular responses →

Thromboxanes Leukotrienes Platelet activating factor | Oxidants | Kinins complement | Cytokines TNF, IL1, IL6, IL8

→ **Inflammation / Vascular Organ System Injury**

Endothelial injury ⟹ Coagulation system activation ⟹ Consumption of protein C

Apoptosis ⟺ Coagulopathy/DIC ⟺ Uncontrolled inflammation

Multi-organ failure → Death

The Three Phases of Shock

Early or Compensated

The early or compensated stage of shock can easily be missed since the animal appears essentially normal. This stage occurs as a result of the baroreceptor-mediated release of catecholamines.

With the development of hypoperfusion of tissues and organs associated with circulatory compromise, baroreceptors in the aortic and carotid arteries detect a decrease in cardiac output and a neural signal is transmitted to the vasomotor center of the medulla oblongata. The baroreceptors increase sympathetic neural activity, which increases the concentration of circulating catecholamines, which stimulates renin release via B1-adrenergic receptors on granular cells of the juxtaglomerular apparatus in the kidney (**Part A**). Epinephrine increases heart rate, cardiac contractility, and systemic vascular resistance through vasoconstriction and decreases blood flow to the gastrointestinal tract, muscle, and skin to maintain adequate flow to the brain and the heart. The heart rate is a key indicator of compensatory shock.

The release of renin in response to the baroreceptor-mediated neural activity activates angiotensin. Angiotensin II works on the adrenal gland to increase secretion of aldosterone from the zona glomerulosa of the adrenal cortex. Aldosterone acts at the cortical collecting duct to reabsorb sodium chloride and water. Angiotensin II is also a strong vasoconstrictor, especially in the gut, causing an increase in blood pressure. Angiotensin II facilitates the release of norepinephrine from the adrenal medulla and sympathetic nervous terminals, which causes an increase in heart rate and contractility and vasoconstriction. In combination, these effects further enhance the attempted restoration of blood pressure and tissue perfusion, increased cardiac performance, and maximal venous return in the face of shock.

Decompensatory Stage

Organ-associated Manifestations The second stage of shock is referred to as middle or early decompensatory stage of shock. There is a sustained reduction and an uneven distribution in blood flow to the kidneys, splanchnic areas, skin, and muscles. Capillary and microcirculatory pooling tends to occur as a result of opening of vascular beds whose capillaries are normally closed. This occurs when precapillary sphincters lose tone and it contributes to the loss of effective circulating blood volume. Vasodilators involved in this process can include histamine, adenosine, ATP, ADP, K+, H+, and nitric oxide (**Part B**).

A decrease in blood supply to the pancreas causes release of the myocardial depressant factor. Myocardial depressant factor acts as a negative cardiac inotrope, predisposes the heart to cardiac arrhythmias, stimulates hepatic venoconstriction, and depresses the reticuloendothelial system.

Persistent hypoperfusion to the gut is thought to be a predisposing factor to cytokine production resulting in multiple organ failure (MOF) and death from shock injury. The gut mucosal barrier function becomes impaired and this allows for bacterial translocation to occur. Recent studies have implicated the gut as a cytokine-generating organ after hypoperfusion injury and that gut-associated bacteria may play an important role in this inflammatory response. Apoptotic loss of intestinal cells may compromise bowel wall integrity and be a mechanism for bacterial or endotoxin translocation into the systemic circulation.

Cellular-associated Manifestations With sustained hypoperfusion, oxygen consumption in tissues becomes dependent on oxygen delivery (DO_2) and anaerobic metabolism, which causes lactic acidosis. Intracellular acidosis leads to the release of lysosomal hydrolases causing release of vasoactive peptides. Capillary endothelial acidosis increases capillary permeability. Acidosis leads to cellular swelling with loss of extracellular fluid volume into the cells. Cellular swelling occurs due to decreased adenosine triphosphate (ATP)-dependent sodium-potassium exchange, which increases intracellular sodium and water concentrations. As lactic acidosis progresses, cellular integrity is lost (**Part C**).

Low oxygen levels can stimulate cellular production of tumor necrosis factor (TNF), interleukin (IL)-1, and IL-8. Inflammatory cytokines play a major role in the development and maintenance of shock.

In cells experiencing sublethal hypoxia, multiple physiologic changes are occurring to alter cellular function and cellular resistance to further injury. This has been termed "hypoxic priming." Intracellular calcium levels increase after cellular hypoxia due to increased permeability of calcium channels. Calcium activates phospholipase, with subsequent release of free fatty acids from cell and organelle membranes. This activates the arachidonic acid cascade. The influx of calcium also activates endogenous cellular proteases facilitating the conversion of xanthine dehydrogenase (XD) to xanthine oxidase (XO). When oxygen is reintroduced into this low-flow system, causing reperfusion, hypoxanthine is oxidized by XO to form superoxide anion radicals, hydrogen peroxide, and hydroxyl anions (see **Part C**).

The reactive oxygen species (ROS) within the cell may damage cell and organelle membranes, denature proteins, and disrupt the chromosomes. Oxidants may also escape from cells, and injure adjacent cells as well as enter the circulation. Endothelial cells in the microvasculature are particularly affected by ROS, which causes microcirculatory disruption. The damaged endothelial cells activate the clotting cascade and support a prothrombotic state, which initiates microvascular thrombosis or disseminated intravascular coagulation (DIC). A number of mechanisms contribute to microvascular compromise including capillary sludging of blood, circulating bacterial toxins, thromboplastin release, acidosis, and activation of complement can all contribute to a hypercoagulable state. As clotting factors are consumed, this can eventually result in a combination of clotting deficits and a consumptive coagulopathy.

Damaged endothelial cells also demonstrate enhanced vascular permeability, resulting in capillary leak phenomena and the development of interstitial space edema and inflammatory mediated cellular injury. This occurs as a result of induced nitric oxide production and the fact that damaged endothelial cells are chemo-attractant and "sticky," facilitating leukocyte adhesion, activation, and migration.

The cumulative effects of the aforementioned processes perpetuate the decompensatory phase of shock by further enhancing hypoperfusion and limiting oxygen delivery.

Terminal Shock

The final stage is termed terminal shock, which is commonly not responsive to aggressive resuscitative therapy. At this stage the intrinsic compensatory mechanisms no longer provide minimal requirements for tissue oxygen delivery and the heart and brain begin to fail under severe tissue hypoxia (**Part D**). Heart rate slows, vasodilation occurs, and blood pools, further reducing blood volume and cardiac output to critical levels. The sustained and overwhelming decrease in perfusion to the myocardium no longer allows the myocardium to maintain cardiac output. The pathophysiology is the same as described for the decompensatory state, except the damage has overwhelmed the body's natural protective mechanisms. Nitric oxide appears to play a major role in the end stages of shock when vascular tone is unresponsive to vasoconstrictor substances and/or therapies. Multiorgan failure occurs and cardiopulmonary arrest is the common sequela.

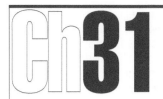

Shock II: Clinical Presentation and Treatment

James Ross, Robert J. Murtaugh, and Kari Moore

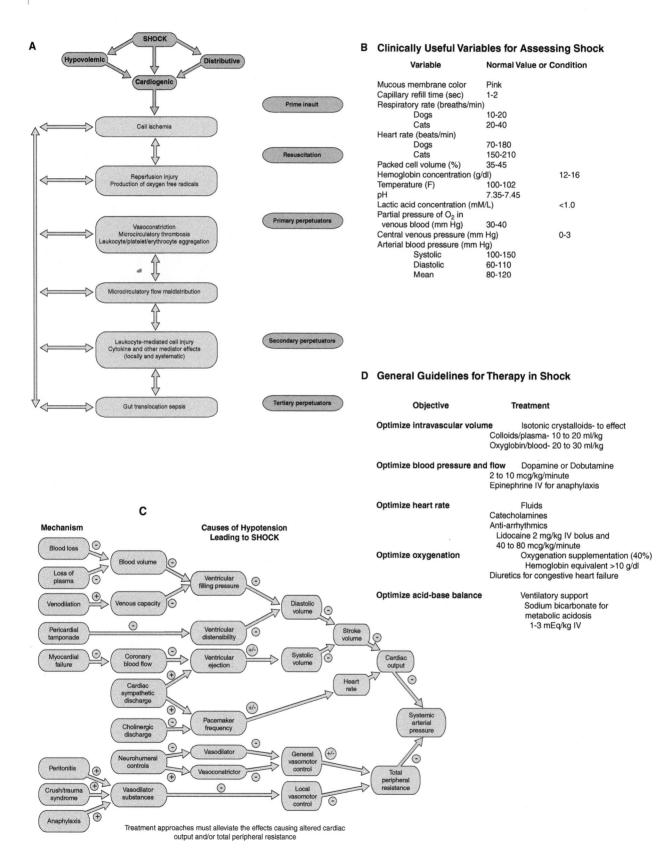

A

B Clinically Useful Variables for Assessing Shock

Variable	Normal Value or Condition	
Mucous membrane color	Pink	
Capillary refill time (sec)	1-2	
Respiratory rate (breaths/min)		
Dogs	10-20	
Cats	20-40	
Heart rate (beats/min)		
Dogs	70-180	
Cats	150-210	
Packed cell volume (%)	35-45	
Hemoglobin concentration (g/dl)		12-16
Temperature (F)	100-102	
pH	7.35-7.45	
Lactic acid concentration (mM/L)		<1.0
Partial pressure of O_2 in venous blood (mm Hg)	30-40	
Central venous pressure (mm Hg)		0-3
Arterial blood pressure (mm Hg)		
Systolic	100-150	
Diastolic	60-110	
Mean	80-120	

D General Guidelines for Therapy in Shock

Objective	Treatment
Optimize intravascular volume	Isotonic crystalloids- to effect Colloids/plasma- 10 to 20 ml/kg Oxyglobin/blood- 20 to 30 ml/kg
Optimize blood pressure and flow	Dopamine or Dobutamine 2 to 10 mcg/kg/minute Epinephrine IV for anaphylaxis
Optimize heart rate	Fluids Catecholamines Anti-arrhythmics Lidocaine 2 mg/kg IV bolus and 40 to 80 mcg/kg/minute
Optimize oxygenation	Oxygenation supplementation (40%) Hemoglobin equivalent >10 g/dl Diuretics for congestive heart failure
Optimize acid-base balance	Ventilatory support Sodium bicarbonate for metabolic acidosis 1-3 mEq/kg IV

Treatment approaches must alleviate the effects causing altered cardiac output and/or total peripheral resistance

Shock occurs when compensatory mechanisms fail to maintain sufficient arterial blood pressure to provide adequate blood flow to organs and tissues. Shock is a state of inadequate tissue perfusion resulting from failure to compensate for one or more of the following: 1) inadequate blood volume, 2) inadequate cardiac pump, and 3) inadequate vascular tone to regulate pressure and flow. Shock is defined at the cellular level as the inadequate delivery of oxygen to the cells of the body as oxygen is the only nutrient that cells cannot store in any appreciable quantity.

Shock is often classified as hypovolemic, cardiogenic, or vasculogenic (distributive) depending on which of these three circulatory system abnormalities was primarily responsible for inadequate tissue perfusion and oxygen delivery (**Part A**). While classifying shock due to major circulatory disorder is helpful in understanding the syndrome, shock is also often described by the disease precipitating the syndrome such as hemorrhagic shock, septic shock, anaphylactic shock, cardiogenic shock, and neurogenic shock. Knowledge of the cause can be helpful in initiating treatment, and each cause of shock may have some distinguishing clinical signs or diagnostic features.

Clinical Presentation

The classic signs for recognition of an animal with decompensatory shock include tachycardia (cats may not exhibit tachycardia), tachypnea, weak pulses due to reduced pulse pressure, an elevated pulse rate, hypothermia with cold skin and limbs as well as pallor of the mucous membranes, a delayed capillary refill time, pupillary dilatation, oliguria, muscle weakness, and a depressed sensorium (**Part B**). Many of these classic clinical signs are due to the compensatory mechanisms that are attempting to restore blood pressure and cardiac output toward normal. Blood pressure in shock is classically low.

The clinical signs associated with the terminal phase of shock are bradycardia with low cardiac output, severe hypotension, pale or cyanotic mucous membranes, absent capillary refill time, weak or absent pulses, severe hypothermia, anuric renal failure, pulmonary edema, and coma.

Cardiogenic shock is differentiated from the other types of shock with a distinguishing feature of distended jugular veins and elevated central venous pressure.

Treatment

With hypovolemic shock, loss of circulating blood volume is a precipitating cause and is the main deficit that must be corrected with treatment. Treatment is indicated for replacing the blood volume with aggressive administration of colloids, crystalloids, and/or blood. The classic clinical findings of shock are generally present and this loss of fluid can result from a variety of mechanisms including internal or external hemorrhage, excessive fluid loss "third-spacing" from inflammatory conditions such as trauma, pancreatitis, or sepsis (**Part C**).

Causes of *cardiogenic shock* include cardiac tamponade, tension pneumothorax, ruptured chordae tendinae, cardiac dysrhythmias, myocardial depression due to toxins and/or myocardial disease, acute pulmonary hypertension or thromboembolism, and/or acute myocardial infarction. *Reduced cardiac output from compromised preload or myocardial performance* is the main cause of the hypotension leading to the cascade of events, and many causes of cardiogenic shock are accompanied by congestive heart failure and signifi-

cant fluid retention. This is an important feature from a therapeutic perspective as fluid therapy (used in all other forms of shock) must be restricted in these individuals with concurrent cardiogenic shock and heart failure.

Anaphylactic shock is classically an allergic phenomenon creating a systemic form of immediate hypersensitivity reaction. Some substance causes a response mediated by IgE, and this results in the release of potent vasodilatory substances by mast cells and basophils (including a lot of histamine) that results in vasodilatation, bronchoconstriction, and activation of the complement and coagulation cascades. Often, the vasodilatation leads to a precipitous drop in blood pressure, edema, laryngeal swelling and upper airway obstruction, reduced pulmonary gas exchange, and eventually hypovolemic shock. *Epinephrine administration* along with fluid resuscitation is required to alleviate the effects of anaphylactic shock. The venous dilatation increases vascular capacity while arterial dilatation and hypotension with reduced venous return are contributing factors in the development of hypovolemia and hypotension. In anaphylactic shock, hypotension, vomiting, diarrhea, ataxia, prostration, coma, and even death can occur within hours if not treated.

In *neurogenic shock,* there is an abrupt loss of vasomotor tone causing a marked increase in vascular capacity and pooling initially within the vascular system which results in a marked decrease in blood pressure and a loss in an "effective" circulating blood volume. Neurogenic shock can be the result of deep anesthesia, spinal anesthesia, spinal cord or central nervous system trauma, prolonged ischemia, or depression of the vasomotor centers, and it is sometimes recognized because bradycardia rather than tachycardia may be present when there is increased intracranial pressure. Treatment must include *attention to the underlying neurologic disease processes such as alleviation of increased intracranial pressure* to ensure adequate resuscitation from neurogenic shock.

In treating shock regardless of cause, keep in mind that shock is a dynamic multisystemic disorder with rapidly changing parameters. Therapy must be dictated by the response to therapy and by monitored parameters. The best monitoring system is the trained clinician's hand on the patient! It is much better to practice prevention than a cure for shock. This means providing for adequate oxygenation, adequate venous return and blood volume, and the management of sepsis and contamination. The basic aims of therapy are to remove the inciting cause, to improve cardiac output and restore circulating blood volume, and to restore the integrity of the microcirculation.

The Future

In addition to traditional therapies for restoring adequate tissue perfusion and oxygen delivery such as aggressive fluid therapy, elimination of cardiac tamponade, or catecholamine administration (**Part D**), the future of treatment options for many shock conditions will likely include administration of substances that will block, blunt, or balance the effects of the mediators of shock and the accompanying coagulation system activation and provide for enhanced cytoprotection from the sequelae of the effects of decreased oxygen delivery. Anti-cytokine therapies, endothelial cell protectants, activated forms of depleted substances such as Protein C, treatments aimed at balancing the beneficial versus the detrimental effects of nitric oxide, and techniques for limiting apoptotic cell death will likely join the armamentarium of options in the treatment of shock.

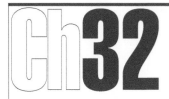

Pathophysiology of Sepsis

Ann Marie Manning

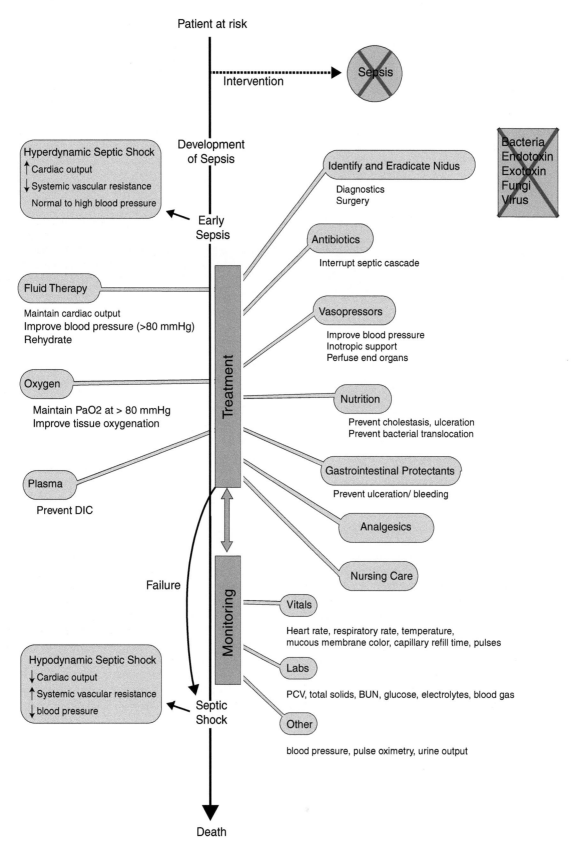

Patient at risk

Intervention → Sepsis ⊗

Bacteria
Endotoxin
Exotoxin
Fungi
Virus

Development
of Sepsis

Identify and Eradicate Nidus

Diagnostics
Surgery

Hyperdynamic Septic Shock
↑ Cardiac output
↓ Systemic vascular resistance
Normal to high blood pressure

Early
Sepsis

Antibiotics

Interrupt septic cascade

Vasopressors

Improve blood pressure
Inotropic support
Perfuse end organs

Fluid Therapy

Maintain cardiac output
Improve blood pressure (>80 mmHg)
Rehydrate

Nutrition

Prevent cholestasis, ulceration
Prevent bacterial translocation

Oxygen

Maintain PaO2 at > 80 mmHg
Improve tissue oxygenation

Gastrointestinal Protectants

Prevent ulceration/ bleeding

Plasma

Prevent DIC

Treatment

Analgesics

Nursing Care

Failure

Monitoring

Vitals

Heart rate, respiratory rate, temperature,
mucous membrane color, capillary refill time, pulses

Hypodynamic Septic Shock
↓ Cardiac output
↑ Systemic vascular resistance
↓ blood pressure

Septic
Shock

Labs

PCV, total solids, BUN, glucose, electrolytes, blood gas

Other

blood pressure, pulse oximetry, urine output

Death

Sepsis and septic shock are frequent and serious problems facing those who treat critically ill veterinary patients. The incidence of sepsis is increasing and is likely due to several factors, including the use of broad-spectrum drugs, evolving resistant organisms, invasive monitoring, and the use of immunosuppressive drugs for the treatment of neoplasia and immune-mediated diseases. Despite aggressive treatment and monitoring, the mortality rate remains as high as 40%–60%.

Terminology is often confusing but the following definitions have been agreed upon by the American College of Chest Physicians and the Society of Critical Care Medicine and have been adapted for use by veterinarians. *Infection* is an inflammatory response secondary to the presence of microorganisms or the invasion of normally sterile tissue by microorganisms. *Bacteremia* is the presence of viable bacteria in the blood. The *systemic inflammatory response syndrome (SIRS)* is the presence of 2 or more of the following conditions regardless of cause (adapted for the cat and dog):

1. Temperature >103 or <100°F
2. Heart rate >140–160 bpm (dog) or >200–220 bpm (cat)
3. Respiratory rate >28 bpm or $PaCO_2$ <32 mm Hg
4. White blood cell count >12,000µL or <4,000µL or ≥10% bands

Sepsis is the SIRS resulting from an infection manifested by 2 or more of the above conditions, but with a clearly documented inciting infectious process. *Sepsis-induced hypotension* is a systolic blood pressure <90 mm Hg or a reduction of >40 mm Hg from baseline in the absence of other causes of hypotension. *Septic shock* is sepsis-induced hypotension despite adequate fluid resuscitation along with the presence of perfusion abnormalities or organ dysfunction. *Multiple-organ dysfunction syndrome (MODS)* is the deterioration of multiple organ systems during SIRS.

Sepsis and Septic Shock

Bacteremia and sepsis are complications of what begins as a local infection. The **Figure** illustrates the sequence of events in the initiation of sepsis and its progression to end-organ dysfunction.

Endotoxin, a lipopolysaccharide (LPS), is found on the cell membrane surface of all gram-negative organisms. LPS is composed of 3 components: the lipid A portion, the core, and an O-specific side chain. The LPS binds to receptors on mononuclear lymphocytes (macrophages and monocytes) and vascular endothelium and results in the secretion of several cytokines from mononuclear cells. The most important of these cytokines are tumor necrosis factor (TNF) and interleukin (IL)-1, which have direct and indirect effects on all organ systems through initiation and amplification of other cytokines.

TNF and IL-1 exert the following direct effects: change temperature set-point (fever induction and hypothermia), decrease vascular resistance, increase vascular permeability, depress cardiac and inotropic function, affect the bone marrow (increase white blood cell count, etc.), cause release of myocardial depressant factor (MDF), and have effects on various enzymes such as lipoprotein lipase and lactate dehydrogenase, which adversely affect energy utilization by tissues. TNF and IL-1 activate complement and kinin cascades and stimulate the production of other cytokines [IL-6, IL-8, IL-10, and platelet-activating factor (PAF)], causing a cascade effect with amplification of these systems. Activation of these secondary mediators initiates the cascade of events leading to derangements in cardiac hemodynamics, systemic oxygen delivery, and pulmonary gas exchange.

Early Versus Late Sepsis

The early systemic effects of sepsis are characterized by a high cardiac output, low systemic vascular resistance, and normal to increased systemic blood pressure. This state is referred to as warm or *hyperdynamic septic shock.* High cardiac output is often maintained despite a decreased ejection fraction caused by circulating MDF. Clinical indicators of hyperdynamic septic shock include fever, tachycardia, tachypnea, brick-red or muddy mucous membranes, hypotension, a decreased arterial-venous oxygen (A-VO$_2$) difference, hypoglycemia, and metabolic acidosis. As the mediators of sepsis continue their effects, cardiac function is depressed further, shunting and capillary leak develop, and blood pressure decreases. These changes may be refractory to fluid therapy, inotropic agents, and vasopressors and characterize the later systemic effects of sepsis described as cold or *hypodynamic septic shock.* Clinical findings associated with hypodynamic septic shock include hypothermia, tachycardia, tachypnea, pallor of mucous membranes, severe hypotension, increased A-VO$_2$ difference, marked mental depression, and possibly bloody diarrhea and evidence of disseminated intravascular coagulation (DIC). If the patient does not respond to therapy during hypodynamic septic shock, death ensues. Death may be the direct result of severe hypotension or may be due to organ failure secondary to hypoperfusion.

Organ Dysfunction During Sepsis-Induced Hypoperfusion

All organ systems are affected by hypoperfusion.

Cardiovascular: As tissue perfusion decreases, sludging of red blood cells occurs and contributes to the generation of microthrombi. Unlike MDF-induced myocardial depression and dilatation, myocardial damage secondary to hypoperfusion is irreversible.

Musculoskeletal: Reduced blood flow to the muscles results in a change from aerobic to anaerobic metabolism, with resulting lactic acid production, metabolic acidosis, and eventually cell death.

Gastrointestinal: Decreased circulation to the abdominal viscera results in a loss of intestinal mucosal integrity and subsequent translocation of GI flora into the bloodstream. Bacterial translocation from compromised intestine contributes to ongoing endotoxemia.

Hepatic: The underperfused liver is similarly affected and is unable to remove bacteria and toxins from the circulation.

Renal: Prerenal acute renal failure or medullary washout with inability to conserve fluid can result from hypoperfusion.

Pulmonary: Poor perfusion results in ventilation-perfusion (V/Q) mismatch. Cytokines and endotoxins produce endothelial damage leading to pulmonary edema, additional V/Q mismatch, and eventually, adult respiratory distress syndorme (ARDS). Edema, V/Q mismatch, and ARDS produce hypoxemia. Because the later stages of sepsis produce irreversible hemodynamic and cardiovascular changes, early recognition and intervention are crucial to a successful outcome for the patient.

Ch33 Diagnosis and Treatment of Sepsis

Ann Marie Manning

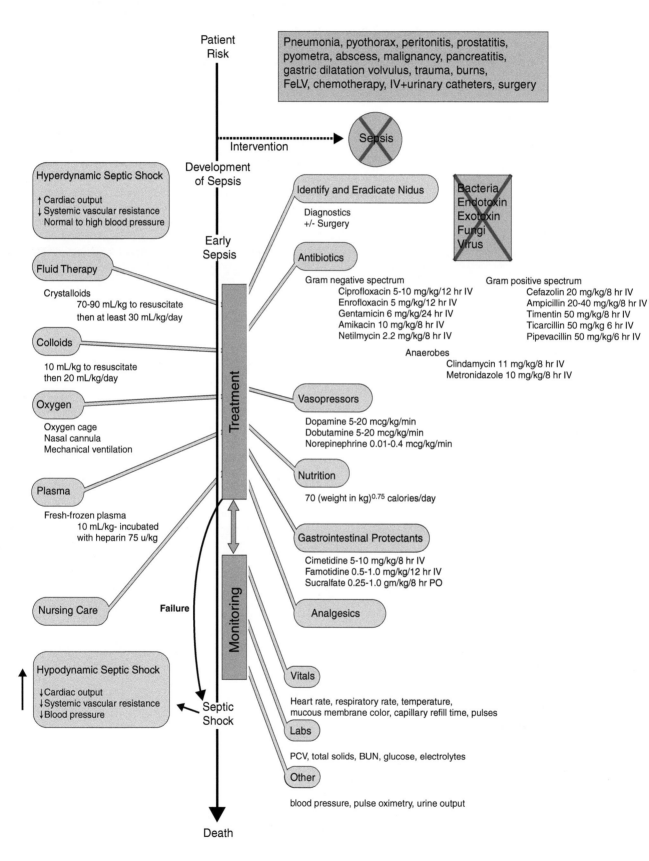

Patient Risk

Pneumonia, pyothorax, peritonitis, prostatitis, pyometra, abscess, malignancy, pancreatitis, gastric dilatation volvulus, trauma, burns, FeLV, chemotherapy, IV+urinary catheters, surgery

Intervention → Sepsis

Development of Sepsis

Identify and Eradicate Nidus

Diagnostics
+/- Surgery

Bacteria
Endotoxin
Exotoxin
Fungi
Virus

Hyperdynamic Septic Shock
↑ Cardiac output
↓ Systemic vascular resistance
Normal to high blood pressure

Early Sepsis

Antibiotics

Gram negative spectrum
Ciprofloxacin 5-10 mg/kg/12 hr IV
Enrofloxacin 5 mg/kg/12 hr IV
Gentamicin 6 mg/kg/24 hr IV
Amikacin 10 mg/kg/8 hr IV
Netilmycin 2.2 mg/kg/8 hr IV

Gram positive spectrum
Cefazolin 20 mg/kg/8 hr IV
Ampicillin 20-40 mg/kg/8 hr IV
Timentin 50 mg/kg/8 hr IV
Ticarcillin 50 mg/kg 6 hr IV
Pipevacillin 50 mg/kg/6 hr IV

Anaerobes
Clindamycin 11 mg/kg/8 hr IV
Metronidazole 10 mg/kg/8 hr IV

Fluid Therapy

Crystalloids
70-90 mL/kg to resuscitate
then at least 30 mL/kg/day

Colloids

10 mL/kg to resuscitate
then 20 mL/kg/day

Treatment

Vasopressors

Dopamine 5-20 mcg/kg/min
Dobutamine 5-20 mcg/kg/min
Norepinephrine 0.01-0.4 mcg/kg/min

Oxygen

Oxygen cage
Nasal cannula
Mechanical ventilation

Nutrition

$70 \text{ (weight in kg)}^{0.75}$ calories/day

Plasma

Fresh-frozen plasma
10 mL/kg- incubated
with heparin 75 u/kg

Gastrointestinal Protectants

Cimetidine 5-10 mg/kg/8 hr IV
Famotidine 0.5-1.0 mg/kg/12 hr IV
Sucralfate 0.25-1.0 gm/kg/8 hr PO

Nursing Care

Failure

Monitoring

Analgesics

Vitals

Heart rate, respiratory rate, temperature, mucous membrane color, capillary refill time, pulses

Hypodynamic Septic Shock
↓ Cardiac output
↓ Systemic vascular resistance
↓ Blood pressure

← Septic Shock

Labs

PCV, total solids, BUN, glucose, electrolytes

Other

blood pressure, pulse oximetry, urine output

Death

The diagnosis of sepsis is based on clinical findings, identification of a septic focus, and laboratory findings. Because of the high morbidity and mortality associated with sepsis and septic shock, prevention is the best treatment. The role of the veterinary clinician therefore is to recognize high-risk patients and to initiate aggressive preventative treatment and monitoring (**Figure**).

Patients at Risk

Patients considered to be at high risk for sepsis include, but are not limited to, those with 1) localized bacterial diseases; 2) debilitating disease—malignancy, pancreatitis, trauma, or burns; 3) immunosuppression—cancer chemotherapy, or corticosteroid therapy; 4) IV or urinary catheters; or 5) postoperative patients.

Clinical Findings

Early sepsis is characterized by a high cardiac output, low systemic vascular resistance, and normal to increased blood pressure. Physical exam findings at this stage usually include fever, tachypnea, tachycardia, bounding femoral pulses, bright red mucous membranes, rapid capillary refill time (<1 second), and weakness. As sepsis progresses to septic shock, cardiac output declines, high vascular resistance is present, and hypotension develops. Clinical findings may include tachycardia, weak or thready femoral pulses, tachypnea, hypothermia, mucous membrane pallor, slow capillary refill time (>2 seconds), severe mental depression, weakness, and evidence of organ failure (oliguria, icterus, hypoxemia, edema, etc.).

Laboratory Findings

When one is presented with a potentially septic patient, initial data should be collected: complete blood cell count, biochemistry profile, urinalysis, arterial blood gas, appropriate cultures (blood, urine, joint fluid, peritoneal or pleural fluid), and coagulation profile. Typical findings in the septic patient are as follows:

1. Complete blood cell count: leukocytosis with a left shift or leukopenia, thrombocytopenia
2. Biochemistry profile: variable findings possibly including hypoglycemia, azotemia, hyperbilirubinemia, elevations in AST and ALT, increased serum lactate, electrolyte derangements
3. Urinalysis: Variable findings, possibly including high or low urine specific gravity, bacteriuria, proteinuria, bilirubinuria, casts
4. Arterial blood gas: hypoxemia, metabolic acidosis, respiratory acidosis or alkalosis
5. Coagulation profile: prolonged prothrombin time (PT) and activated partial thromboplastin time (APTT), thrombocytopenia, elevated fibrin split products
6. Cultures: commonly, gram-negative bacteria gram-positive aerobic cocci, and *Enterococcus*.

Treatment

Adequate cellular oxygenation is the goal of all supportive treatment. Treatment is based on support of organ perfusion with IV fluids, colloids, and vasopressors while attempting to interrupt the progression of sepsis by identifying the septic focus and administering antibiotics.

The *nidus* or source of infection should be identified as quickly as possible, and attempts should be made to drain, debride, or remove the focus surgically. In order to direct antibiotic therapy, cultures should be taken from appropriate sites when the source is identified (urine, joint, peritoneal or pleural cavity, abscesses, etc). If a source cannot be identified, as is the case in 20%–30% of patients, blood and urine cultures should be obtained.

Antibiotic therapy is the backbone of treatment in septic patients. Broad-spectrum antibiotic therapy should be instituted as soon as sepsis is suspected and then refined on the basis of culture results. Initial antibiotic choices should have spectrum against gram-positive and -negative organisms as well as anaerobes. A β-lactam antibiotic

aminoglycoside, and metronidazole represent a good, initial combination. As killed bacteria release endotoxin from their cell walls, the patient should receive adequate fluid and cardiac support prior to antibiotic therapy.

Hemodynamic Support

If the patient is in shock, an initial IV fluid bolus (lactated Ringer's or isotonic saline solution) should be administered at 90 mL/kg (dog) and 70 mL/kg (cat). The initial bolus of crystalloids may be reduced by 40% and administered in conjunction with a colloid such as oxyglobin hetastarch or dextran 70 (10 mL/kg). Following fluid resuscitation, colloids may be used at a rate of 20 mL/kg/day in conjunction with crystalloids. Maintenance fluid therapy requires individual assessment of ongoing losses and the patient's mean arterial blood pressure.

If optimal fluid balance does not maintain blood pressure in the desired range, then a *vasopressor* should be utilized. Dopamine (5–20 μg/kg/min) is the first drug of choice because it possesses both vasopressor and inotropic effects and helps to maintain kidney perfusion. If dopamine alone is inadequate, norepinephrine (0.01–0.4 μg/kg/min) for increased vasopressor support or dobutamine (5–20 μg/kg/min) for inotropic support may be added. Patients on elevated doses of these drugs require ECG monitoring as arrhythmias may occur. Unresponsiveness to vasopressor support indicates a poor prognosis.

Oxygen Therapy

Supplemental oxygen should be administered to septic patients to maximize oxygen delivery to the tissues. Sepsis causes a maldistribution of blood flow, resulting in intraorgan shunting and cellular death. Hypoxemia is common due to ventilation-perfusion mismatch from decreased perfusion and interstitial and alveolar edema. Attempts should be made to maintain the patient's $PaO_2 > 80$ mmHg. To maximize oxygen delivery to the tissues in anemic patients, packed red blood cells should be administered to maintain the hematocrit at a minimum of 25%.

Nutrition and Miscellaneous Therapies

Sepsis produces a hypermetabolic state that should be supported with adequate nutrition.

Patients whose blood glucose is <70 gm/dL should receive a slow IV bolus of 50% dextrose (1 mL/kg) diluted 1:1 with saline. Dextrose may then be added to daily IV fluids to produce a 2.5%–5.0% solution. Animals with evidence of DIC may receive fresh-frozen plasma (10 mL/kg) incubated with heparin (75 U/kg incubated 30 minutes prior to administration). Gastric protectants such as sucralfate (0.25–1.00 gm PO every 8 hours), cimetidine (5–8 mg/kg IV every 8 hours), or famotidine (0.5–1.00 mg/kg IV every 12 hours) may be used for GI bleeding.

Monitoring

Septic patients should be monitored carefully as sepsis is a continuum that produces minute-to-minute changes in the patient's condition that require continuous treatment adjustments. Monitoring should include daily evaluation of packed cell volume, total solids, blood glucose, electrolytes, blood gas, urine output, and blood pressure. Heart rate, respiratory rate, body temperature, mucous membrane color, capillary refill time, and pulse quality should be checked regularly.

Future Directions

New treatments for sepsis are constantly evolving and are aimed at interrupting the inflammatory pathways. Currently inhibitors of nitric oxide synthase, platelet-activating factor antagonists, endogenous opiate antagonists, cyclooxygenase inhibitors, and monoclonal antibodies are being investigated.

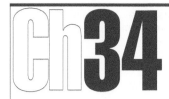

Coagulation System/Physiology

Kari Moore

A Primary Coagulation

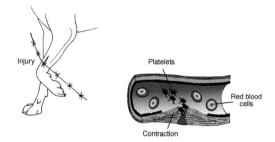

B Secondary Clot

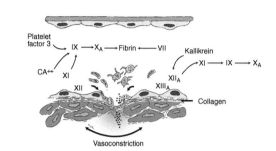

C Fibrinolysis

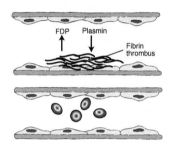

D Coagulation Tests

Prothrombin time: V, VII, X, II, I
Partial thromboplastin time: XII, XI, IX,VIII,X, V, II, I
Vitamin K-responsive factors: II, VII, IX, X
Abbreviated clotting cascade:

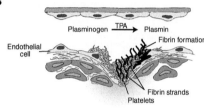

E

Factor	Breeds Affected	Bleeding Time	PT	PTT	ACT	Definitive Test
von Willerbrands	Doberman pinscher, Airdales, Shetland sheepdog Reported in many dog breeds	A	N	Variable	Variable	Low VIII Low VIII-related antigen
VIII	Reported in many dog and cat breeds	N	N	A	A	Low VIII; N to increased VIII-related antigen
IX	Reported in many dog and cat breeds	N	N	A	A	Low IX
VII	Beagle, Alaskan Malamute	N	A	N	N	Low VII, normal RVVT
XI	Springer spaniel, Great Pyrenees	N	N	A	A	Low XI
XII	Domestic cat	N	N	A	A	Low XII
X	Cocker spaniel	N	A	A	A	Low X, abnormal RVVT

A= abnormal
N= normal
RVVT= Russell viper venom time

The normal coagulation system is a finely tuned process designed to prevent both significant hemorrhage and intravascular thrombosis. The 3 main events that surround clot formation are primary hemostasis, secondary hemostasis, and fibrinolysis. This chapter discusses these main events and the clinical findings in coagulopathies as well as diagnostic tests to document specific coagulopathies.

Primary Hemostasis

A primary clot is formed when the vascular wall is damaged. (**Part A**). Injured arterioles and venules respond by contraction of the smooth muscle within their walls. This response lasts approximately 60 seconds, but it does help to decrease the hydrostatic pressure and subsequent blood flow, in order for the platelets to adhere to the exposed surface. A normal primary clot formation depends on an adequate number of platelets and normal platelet function. Platelets are formed from megakaryocytes in the bone marrow and have a life span of about 10 days, with 30% of the platelets stored in the spleen. After adhesion occurs, there is platelet-platelet adhesion, which is termed *aggregation*. The growth of the platelet aggregate is halted by flowing blood. The platelet aggregation provides a temporary hemostatic seal for coagulation proteins to form a more permanent clot.

Secondary Clot

Secondary hemostasis combines the primary aggregated platelet plug with the coagulation proteins to form a fibrin clot (**Part B**). The coagulation cascade has been divided into the intrinsic, extrinsic, and common pathways. These pathways are interrelated. All the coagulation proteins except factor VIII are produced by the liver. Factor VIII is produced by vascular endothelial cells and by megakaryocytes.

The intrinsic pathway begins when factor XII is exposed to collagen or a subendothelial surface. Prekallikrein and high-molecular-weight kininogen are 2 of the factors that regulate the rate of factor XII activation. When factor XII becomes surface bound, a conformational change takes place, making the molecule more susceptible to proteolytic cleavage by plasma kallikrein. Kallikrein stimulates the kinin, coagulation, and fibrinolytic systems. Plasma kallikrein converts factor XII to activated factor XII (XIIa). Factor XIIa converts factor XI to XIa, which converts IX to IXa. Factor VIII, calcium, platelet phospholipids, and factor IXa form a complex that converts factor X to Xa.

The extrinsic pathway is made up of 1 factor, factor VII, Factor VII, when combined with tissue thromboplastin, directly activates factor X and IX.

Factor X begins the common pathway. Factor Xa combines with factor Va, calcium, and platelet phospholipids to convert factor II (prothrombin) to factor IIa (thrombin). Thrombin is then the catalyst that converts fibrinogen to fibrin. Thrombin acts as a positive feedback mechanism on factors V, VIII, and XII and on platelets. Fibrin is stabilized by factor XIIIa. Factor XII is activated by thrombin in the presence of calcium.

Fibrinolysis

Fibrinolysis is the breakdown of a formed clot (**Part C**). The major component of the fibrinolytic system is plasminogen. This is the inactive form of plasmin. Plasminogen is converted to plasmin by tissue plasminogen activator (TPA), which is produced by the endothelial cells. The conversion is also induced by factor XIIa and kallikrein. Plasmin works to break down fibrinogen and fibrin. Some of the by-products of this breakdown [Fibrin/fibrinogen degradation products (FDPs)] also work as fibrinolytic agents. After plasmin has reacted locally with fibrinogen or fibrin, it is released back in the plasma and is inactivated by forming complexes with α2-antiplasmin and α2-macroglobulin.

Clinical Relevance

Clinical symptoms of a coagulopathy are hematomas, spontaneous bleeding, shifting lameness due to hemarthrosis, large areas of bruising, and excessive bleeding during and after surgery. This is different from platelet abnormalities where the primary clinical signs are multiple small bruises and spontaneous bleeding from mucosal surfaces, such as epistaxis, hematuria, melena, and gingival bleeding. The von Willebrand disease and DIC can have clinical signs of both, depending on the severity of the disease. Inherited coagulopathies are rare, but do occasionally occur. They are usually recognized after abnormal, recurring bleeding episodes in young animals. Acquired coagulopathies usually are noted in older animals, and it is usually the first time they have presented with a bleeding tendency. A basic coagulation profile, which would include a platelet count, PT, partial thromboplastin time (PTT), fibrinogen level, and FDP measurement, would be performed first as a screening test (**Part D**). The PT tests mainly for the extrinsic pathway and is prolonged with deficiencies in factor V, VII, X, II, or I, but is most sensitive to a factor VII deficiency. Activated PTT tests mainly for the intrinsic pathway and is prolonged with deficiencies in factor XII, XI, IX, VIII, X, V, II, or I. With both of these tests a prolongation or shortening of 25% or greater is a significant finding. An in-house test that can be performed quickly is the activated clotting time (ACT). The ACT results in activation of factor XII and evaluates primarily the intrinsic and common pathways. Prolongation of the ACT usually parallels prolongation of the activated PTT, although in rare instances severe thrombocytopenia can also prolong the ACT. The ACT is usually considered normal if it is <120 seconds in a dog and <90 seconds in a cat. Another in-house test is the bucchal mucosal bleeding time (BMBT). It evaluates the interaction between the platelets and endothelium that lead to the formation of a primary hemostatic clot. The BMBT is prolonged mainly in animals with thrombocytopenia or a platelet dysfunction syndrome. Reference values for normal dogs and cats are 1–3 minutes. Based on any abnormalities of these initial tests, more specific factor analysis would be performed if a congenital coagulopathy is suspected. **Part E** shows the factor abnormality, the test abnormalities, and the most common breeds affected.

Two main acquired coagulopathies are vitamin K deficiency, usually due to warfarin-type toxicity, and DIC. DIC is discussed in Chapter 35. Vitamin K–dependent factors are factors II, VII, IX, and X (see **Part D**). The half-lives of the factors are 41, 6, 14, and 16.5 hours, respectively. This explains why the PT will be prolonged sooner than the APTT. Vitamin K deficiency is rare in neonatal puppies and kittens and is usually transient if present. Only a small amount of vitamin K is necessary to sustain adequate synthesis of these factors, which explains why it takes a long time for chronic biliary obstruction, liver disease, and malabsorption syndromes to cause coagulopathies. Vitamin K deficiency is confirmed by history and a prolonged ACT, PT, or PTT. If symptoms are severe, administration of fresh-frozen plasma is necessary along with vitamin K supplementation as initial treatment of the disease. Fresh-frozen plasma will work immediately to replace the vitamin K–deficient factors, until the liver has had time to produce active factors with the vitamin K supplementation. Poisoning with the longer-acting rat poisons, such as broudifacoum, may require vitamin K supplementation for as long as 3–6 weeks.

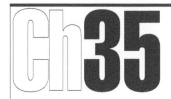

Disseminated Intravascular Coagulopathy

Kari Moore

A   Disseminated Intravascular Coagulation

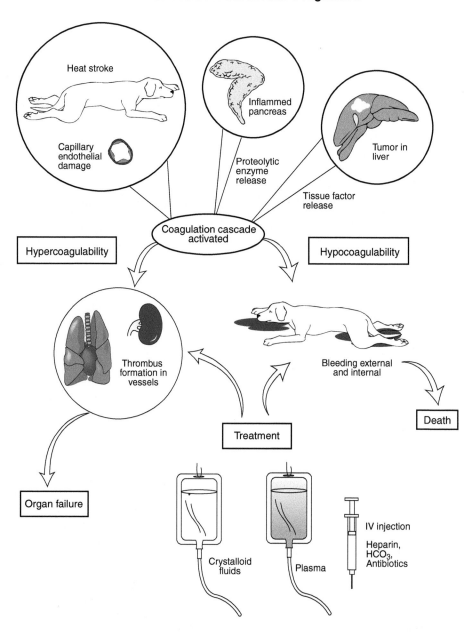

B   Diagnostic Test

Diagnostic Test	Results in DIC
Peripheral blood smear	± Fragmentocytes, thrombocytopenia
Thrombocyte count	Low
Plasma fibrinogen	Usually low, may be normal or high
FDP	Increased
D-Dimers	Increased
PT	Normal or prolonged
APTT	Normal or prolonged
AT III	Normal or low
FM agglutination test	Positive
Thrombin or Reptilase time	Prolonged

DIC is almost always secondary sequela to an underlying disease process. Diseases causing DIC include neoplasia, acute pancreatitis, immune-mediated hemolytic anemia, heatstroke, sepsis, and many others (**Part A**).

Pathogenesis

The clotting cascade is a finely tuned mechanism that controls hemostasis while preventing generalized thrombosis. In DIC, intravascular triggering occurs in excess to disrupt the equilibrium, overwhelm the compensatory mechanisms, and cause uncontrolled thrombosis and/or hemorrhaging.

Normal clot formation is discussed in Chapter 34. What occurs in DIC is an upset of the delicate balance the body has between thrombus formation and fibrinolysis and the ability to keep these processes confined to a localized area. Three ways for the system to be overwhelmed is by DIC-inducing proteolytic enzymes (snake venom), damaged vascular endothelium, or thromboplastic substances that may be released from necrotic tissues or secreted by malignant tumors. (see **Part A**). Any of these will cause an activation of the clotting cascade to produce thrombin. Thrombin will convert fibrinogen to fibrin, which can become trapped in the microcirculation and cause thrombi. Thrombi are not always formed because thrombin will cause fibrinogen to be degraded into small fibrinopeptides and soluble fibrin monomers (FMs). When circulation and the reticuloendothelial system (RES) are normal, the FMs can be eliminated from the blood by the liver, which will prevent fibrin formation. Thrombi formation is also caused by a decrease in antithrombin III (AT III). Low AT III occurs with liver disease, nephrotic syndrome, L-asparaginase therapy, or prolonged heparin administration, or as a hereditary deficiency. DIC thrombus formation is exacerbated by metabolic conditions such as hypoxemia, acidosis, circulatory stasis, and shock (see **Part A**). Hypoxemia causes anaerobic glycolysis, which causes acidosis. Acidosis (metabolic or respiratory) contributes to DIC because low pH inhibits heparin and AT III. Circulatory stasis prevents the removal of fibrin and FDPs and prevents AT III from being supplied to where it is needed. Stasis also can lead to vascular endothelial damage, anoxia, and acidosis of tissue. Shock will enhance DIC for the same reasons as circulatory stasis.

Hemorrhage is more clinically evident in most cases of DIC than is thrombi formation. Hemorrhage is caused when the fibrinolytic system destroys fibrin, fibrinogen, and other clotting factors. Consumption of the coagulation factors and platelets in the clotting process can lead to thrombocytopenia and decreased clotting factors, causing bleeding tendencies. DIC also has a positive feedback mechanism since the (FDPs) inhibit thrombin and interfere with fibrin polymerization. DIC is enhanced with the paralysis of the RES since this will inhibit the removal of FDPs and microthrombi. Decreased AT III creates an environment more likely to induce thrombi formation.

Clinical Presentation

DIC can manifest differently in each patient, owing to the underlying cause, the condition of the patient, and chronicity of the DIC. DIC may be undetected clinically except through laboratory test results (**Part B**). It can present as generalized ecchymoses, petechiae, epistaxis, hematuria, hematechezia, melena, intraocular bleeding, and bleeding from venipuncture sites, surgical sites, and mild trauma. It can cause significant internal bleeding such as a hemothorax or hemoabdomen. Microthrombi can cause clinical signs related to ischemic damage of the kidneys, liver, GI tract, lungs, or CNS. Signs such as dyspnea, acute renal failure, hypovolemic shock, and necrosis of tissue can be seen depending on the affected organ or organs. Thromboemboli occasionally are found in the larger vessels.

Laboratory Diagnosis

Unfortunately, there is no one specific test to determine whether an animal is in DIC. A multitude of tests along with clinical signs must be evaluated to reach a diagnosis. In overt DIC, the diagnosis can be made by a combination of thrombocytopenia and grossly abnormal blood clot formation and lysis. In more subtle cases, multiple tests may need to be evaluated to diagnose DIC.

Peripheral Blood Smear and Platelet Count

This easy in-house test can be used as a starting point. A peripheral blood smear can be used to evaluate for fragmentocytes or shistocytes. Fragmentocytes (see **Part B**) can be seen in DIC because red blood cells that flow through impartial clots formed in the vasculature from DIC can fragment. Severe thrombocytopenia also can be detected on a blood smear. Thrombocytopenia is a hallmark of DIC. A diagnosis of DIC can be ruled out in the presence of persistently normal thrombocyte counts.

Fibrinogen, FDP, and D-Dimer Assays

Plasma fibrinogen concentrations are usually low with DIC, but also may be normal or elevated due to compensatory overproduction in chronic DIC.

In DIC, the FDP concentration should be ≥ 10 µg/mL. The FDP concentration is not an indication of the severity of DIC and can be negative due to low fibrinogen or chronic DIC.

In DIC, the D-Dimer concentration is often moderately to markedly elevated at > 1000 mg/dL. Values of 250–500 mg/dL may be seen "normally" in the postsurgical patient.

PT and Activated PTT (APTT)

The APTT is usually prolonged since many of the factors in the intrinsic and common pathways are consumed in DIC. The PT may also be prolonged, but this is not always the case.

AT III and FMs

Plasma AT III levels were shown to be low in 85% of patients with DIC. This test is not readily available.

The FM agglutination test result is negative in normal dogs and almost always positive in animals with DIC. The blood must be drawn carefully or false-positive findings result from FM formation in vitro owing to thrombin generation.

Thrombin and Reptilase Time

Thrombin and reptilase are fibrinogen-converting enzymes that are inhibited by FDPs. The clotting time of plasma is usually prolonged in DIC patients when thrombin or reptilase is added. Both times are also abnormal if the plasma fibrinogen concentration is <100 mg/mL. Reptilase is beneficial in monitoring the progression or resolution of DIC because heparin does not interfere with the test results.

Therapy

The mainstay of therapy is to treat the underlying disease. When this is not possible, the prognosis is guarded at best. Since it may take some time to determine the underlying cause, it is best to start supportive care (see **Part A**). It is important to treat problems that contribute to DIC, such as shock, hypovolemia, acid-base and electrolyte imbalances, and anemia.

For normovolemic, nonanemic patients with DIC, fresh plasma or fresh-frozen plasma should be given. An IV dose of 10 mL/kg is recommended. This helps to replace many clotting factors and AT III. Fresh or fresh-frozen plasma can be incubated with 75 U of heparin/kg to help enhance the AT III ability in the plasma. Heparin itself does nothing to help with fibrinolysis, but combines with AT III to enhance its effect by 10–1000-fold. The recommended dose of heparin is 75 U/kg SQ every 8 hours. This dose will not affect the APTT allowing for sequential monitoring that reflects resolution, or not, of DIC.

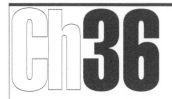

Hypertension

Lisa L. Powell

Hypertension

A Normal Blood Pressure Values (mm Hg)

Canine
- Systolic 120
- Diastolic 80
- Mean 100

Feline
- Systolic 190-200
- Diastolic 140

B Control of Blood Pressure

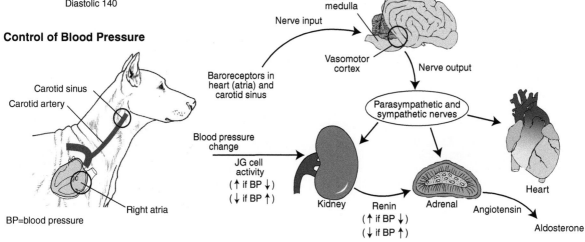

Cerebellum

Pons/medulla

Nerve input

Vasomotor cortex

Nerve output

Baroreceptors in heart (atria) and carotid sinus

Carotid sinus

Carotid artery

Blood pressure change

JG cell activity
(↑ if BP ↓)
(↓ if BP ↑)

Parasympathetic and sympathetic nerves

Heart

Kidney

Renin
(↑ if BP ↓)
(↓ if BP ↑)

Adrenal

Angiotensin

Aldosterone

Right atria

BP=blood pressure

C Causes of Hypertension

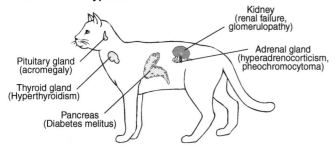

Kidney (renal failure, glomerulopathy)

Adrenal gland (hyperadrenocorticism, pheochromocytoma)

Pituitary gland (acromegaly)

Thyroid gland (Hyperthyroidism)

Pancreas (Diabetes melitus)

D Clinical Signs of Hypertension

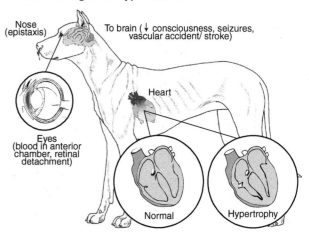

Nose (epistaxis)

To brain (↓ consciousness, seizures, vascular accident/ stroke)

Heart

Eyes (blood in anterior chamber, retinal detachment)

Normal

Hypertrophy

E Indirect Blood Pressure Measurement (Doppler Technique)

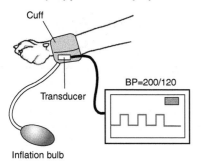

Cuff

BP=200/120

Transducer

Inflation bulb

F Antihypertensive Medications

Drug	Dose
Amlodipine (calcium channel blocker)	Cats: 0.625 mg (1/4 of a 2–mg tab) once daily PO
Enalapril (ACE inhibitor)	Dogs: 0.25–5.55 mg/kg, once–twice daily PO
Sodium nitroprusside (life-threatening hypertension)	Dogs: 2.5–5.0 mg/kg/min Cats: 0.5–2.0 mg/kg/min, IV only
Esmolol (life-threatening hypertension)	Loading: 500 mg/kg CRI: 50 mg/kg/min, IV only
Diuretics, a blockers, b blockers, hydralazine	See specific drugs for doses

Hypertension is defined as a sustained elevation of systolic or diastolic arterial blood pressure above the normal value reported for that species. Blood pressure is determined by cardiac output multiplied by systemic vascular resistance. Cardiac output is measured as heart rate times stroke volume. Stroke volume is determined by cardiac contractility and blood volume. Mean blood pressure is calculated as diastolic pressure plus $\frac{1}{3}$ (systolic minus diastolic pressure). Average normal blood pressures in dogs and cats are shown in **Part A**.

Physiology

Normal blood pressure is controlled through many different mechanisms. The vasomotor center, located in the medulla and pons, contains sympathetic and parasympathetic nerve fibers that control heart rate and contractility. Baroreceptors and chemoreceptors located in the heart and blood vessel walls send impulses to the vasomotor center in response to high and low systemic blood pressure. The renin-angiotensin-aldosterone (RAA) system is a very important mechanism in the control of blood pressure (**Part B**). When arterial blood pressure decreases, the juxtaglomerular cells of the kidneys release renin, an enzyme that converts angiotensinogen to angiotensin I. Angiotensin I is converted to angiotensin II in the lungs by angiotensin-converting enzyme (ACE). Angiotensin II is one of the most potent vasoconstrictors known, thus causing an increase in systemic vascular resistance and therefore systemic blood pressure. Angiotensin II also stimulates the release of aldosterone, causing increased reabsorption of salt and water by the kidneys. This increases circulating plasma volume and contributes to the maintenance of normal blood pressure.

Etiology

There are many causes of hypertension in dogs and cats (**Part C**). The most common cause in both species is renal failure, and the severity of the renal failure does not correlate with the presence or absence of hypertension. Other causes of hypertension in dogs include hyperadrenocorticism, pheochromocytoma, hypothyroidism, and acromegaly. Primary hypertension has been reported in 1 colony of beagles. The 2 most common causes of hypertension in cats are chronic renal failure and hyperthyroidism. Other less common causes include pheochromocytoma and acromegaly. Hyperparathyroidism and diabetes mellitus have been associated with hypertension in people, but has not been reported in animal species. Accidental ingestion of some drugs can cause hypertension in animals.

Renal failure is thought to produce hypertension through several proposed mechanisms, including decreased excretion of salt and water and activation of the RAA system. Hyperthyroidism causes an upregulation of β receptors in the myocardium, causing increased sensitivity to circulating catecholamines. An increase in heart rate, stroke volume, and cardiac output occurs with a resultant increase in systemic blood pressure. Pheochromocytoma causes hypertension through the release of catecholamines from the chromaffin cells of the tumor. Severe blood pressure elevations occur, and signs referable to hypertension may be the presenting clinical complaint.

Clinical Signs

Systemic hypertension most often affects the brain, heart, and kidneys. Clinical features include the following (**Part D**):

CNS deficits from cerebral or brain stem vascular rupture and hemorrhage (i.e., seizures, disorientation, or abnormal behavior)
Epistaxis
Blindness from retinal edema, hemorrhage, and detachments

Left ventricular hypertrophy, systolic heart murmur related to mitral regurgitation, with or without S4 gallop sound (these changes secondary to a sustained increase in afterload with systemic hypertension)
Signs referable to the underlying disease process: PU/PD, polyphagia, weight loss in cats in spite of polyphagia, weight gain in dogs secondary to hypothyroidism

Diagnosis

If systemic hypertension is suspected, blood pressure should be measured. This can be challenging in small animals, owing to movement, small arterial vessel diameter, and false elevations secondary to the stress of being in the hospital. Blood pressure is most often measured using indirect methods. Two methods commonly used are Doppler and oscillometric measurements (**Part E**). The Doppler uses ultrasonic signals to detect changes in arterial pulsations, and a pressure cuff is used to determine systolic and diastolic pressures. It is important to use the correct cuff size for accurate measurements. The cuff size should be 30% of the circumference of the limb. The metatarsal artery or median artery is most often used for Doppler measurements. The oscillometric method of blood pressure measurement is more accurate in dogs because of the larger arterial diameter in this species. The oscillometric technique detects blood flow changes below the inflated cuff as it is occluding the artery. It displays systolic, diastolic, and mean blood pressures. The drawback to this method is an average inaccuracy of 10 mm Hg in blood pressure measurements. A minimum of 3 measurements should be done to obtain an accurate reading.

Treatment

Acute, life-threatening hypertension must be treated immediately to avoid serious end-organ damage. Sodium nitroprusside relaxes both arteries and veins within seconds of the start of infusion and disappears almost as rapidly when the infusion is discontinued. Sodium nitroprusside should be used to bring down arterial blood pressure by 20%–30% (**Part F**). Because of its rapid onset of action and potency, nitroprusside infusion must be monitored closely by means of an infusion pump, and arterial blood pressure must be monitored continuously by either direct or indirect measurements. The main side effect of nitroprusside therapy is severe hypotension and usually is caused by inadequate regulation of the infusion rate, or inadvertent flushing of the IV line containing the nitroprusside solution. The immediate metabolic product of nitroprusside is cyanide. Cyanide poisoning is rare but can occur, especially in cats with decreased ability to convert cyanide to thiocyanate or in patients with significant renal insufficiency. Esmolol, an ultra-short-acting β-blocker (β₁ specific), can also be used as a continuous-rate infusion to treat a hypertensive crisis. Esmolol must be administered at a loading dose, followed by an IV constant-rate infusion (CRI) (see **Part F**).

Long-term control of hypertension can be achieved through several drugs (see **Part F**). Amlodipine, a calcium channel blocker, is very effective in controlling hypertension, especially in cats. Amlodipine should be effective within 24–48 hours. ACE inhibitors are effective in reducing arterial blood pressure through inhibition of the RAA system. Enalapril is most often used in dogs. Salt restriction is helpful in combination with other drugs to reduce intravascular volume, but is often ineffective as the sole means of controlling hypertension.

Treatment of the underlying cause of hypertension can often result in the resolution of systemic blood pressure elevations. Most patients with chronic renal failure require lifelong therapy with antihypertensive medication. Retinal detachments and blindness may not resolve, and seizure activity may continue if a focus was established during a hypertensive crisis.

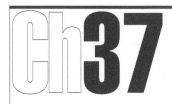

Hyperthermia I: Pathophysiology

Armelle DeLaforcade

A Effect of Hyperthermia on Organ Function

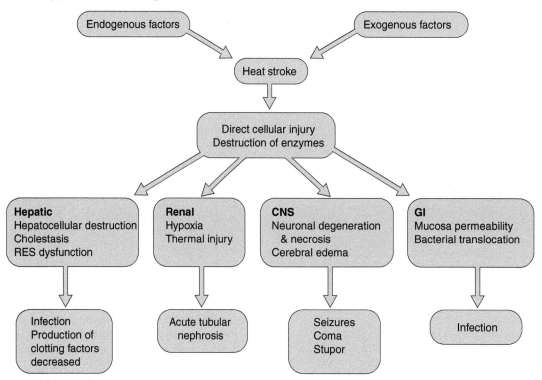

B Effect of Hyperthermia on the Circulatory System

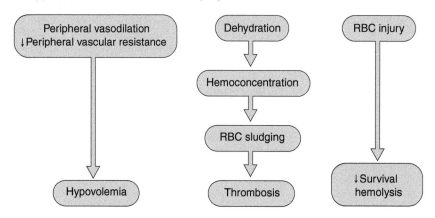

C Effect of Hyperthermia on the Hemostatic System

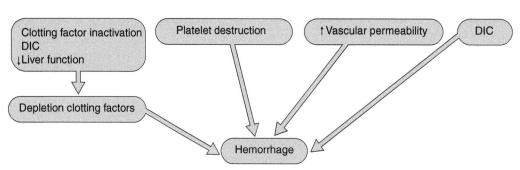

Heatstroke is a frequently encountered disorder in veterinary medicine, particularly in the summer months when hot humid conditions prevail. Heatstroke can be defined as severe hyperthermia resulting in thermal injury to tissues. Nonexertional heatstroke occurs when animals are confined to hot humid environments lacking ventilation. Exertional heatstroke occurs following strenuous activity in hot humid weather. Injuries relating to heatstroke are due to the direct effect of heat on cellular and enzyme function.

Physiology

Under normal circumstances cats and dogs maintain their body temperature over a wide range of environmental temperature variations. The thermoregulatory center is located in the hypothalamus and receives input both from hypothalamic sensor cells which detect the temperature of circulating blood, and cutaneous receptor cells. In response to mild heat stress, reflex vasoactivity occurs which leads to the shunting of blood from muscles and visceral organs to the periphery where subsequent cutaneous vasodilation allows heat loss by radiation and convection. During moderate heat stress, panting provides a means of heat loss by evaporation as large volumes of air move across the mucosa of the oropharynx and tongue.

Heat stroke occurs when these compensatory mechanisms fail or are overwhelmed. Heat stroke must be differentiated from pyrexia. Pyrexia leads to resetting of the thermoregulatory center in response to a pathological process such as infection or inflammation. In contrast to this, heatstroke occurs when the normal thermoregulatory system of the body is overwhelmed by exposure to extreme heat stress.

Predisposing Factors

Factors predisposing to heat stroke include those causing either increased heat production or impaired heat loss (**Part A**). Endogenous factors include pre-existing respiratory or cardiac disease which can cause an animal to become vulnerable to heat stroke by compromising heat dissipation. Abnormalities in the central nervous system (the hypothalamus in particular) can impair the ability to thermoregulate. Extremes in age can also result in thermoregulatory problems, as infants do not acquire the ability to thermoregulate until they are 45 days old. Geriatric patients often have underlying cardiac or respiratory disease which decreases their ability to tolerate heat stress. Obese animals are predisposed to heat stroke due to their tendency to retain heat, and abnormal upper airway conformation leads to difficulties with heat dissipation in brachycephalic breeds.

Exogenous factors include extreme exercise, high humidity, and confinement in poorly ventilated areas. Lack of acclimatization can predispose to heat stress, as can water deprivation. Drugs predisposing to heat stroke include phenothiazine derivatives, and diuretics. Phenothiazines cause disturbances in thermoregulation by depressing the reticular activating system, while diuretics lead to depletion of fluid and electrolytes with subsequent dehydration.

Toxins predisposing to heat stroke include strychnine and organophosphates. Strychnine causes tetanic seizures induced by touch, noise, and bright light which can lead to extreme heat production. Organophosphates are anticholinesterases, and also cause heat production through muscle fasciculations and convulsions in severely affected animals.

Pathophysiology

The damaging effects of heatstroke are due to direct cellular injury and destruction of enzymes. The circulatory system is compromised due to peripheral vasodilation and decreased peripheral vascular resistance leading to hypovolemia. Hemoconcentration due to dehydration can predispose to red blood cell sludging and subsequent thrombosis (**Part B**). Red blood cell injury occurs and results in decreased survival time and hemolysis. The depletion of clotting factors through inactivation, disseminated intravascular coagulation (DIC), as well as decreased production from hepatic injury predisposes the heatstroke patient to hemorrhage. Hemorrhage can also occur as a result of platelet destruction, increases in vascular permeability due to damaged endothelium, and DIC (**Part C**).

Thermal injury of the central nervous system (CNS) results in neuronal degeneration and necrosis. Resulting cerebral edema can lead to stupor, paddling behavior, seizures, and coma.

Hepatic damage due to thermal injury includes hepatocellular destruction, cholestasis, and dysfunction of the hepatic reticuloendothelial system (see **Part A**). Such compromise of immune function along with bacterial translocation due to damaged gastrointestinal mucosa predisposes the heatstroke patient to infection.

The combination of direct thermal injury as well as hypoxia from decreased circulating volume and increased metabolic demand for oxygen predispose the kidneys to acute tubular nephrosis. Rhabdomyolysis resulting in myoglobinuria can also be a contributing factor.

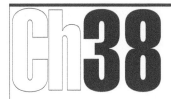

Hyperthermia II: Diagnosis and Treatment

Armelle DeLaforcade

A Effect of Hyperthermia on Organ Function

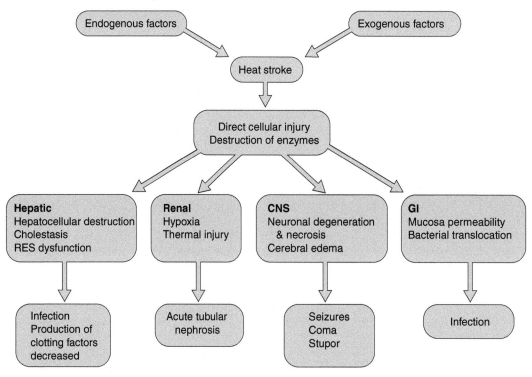

B Effect of Hyperthermia on the Circulatory System

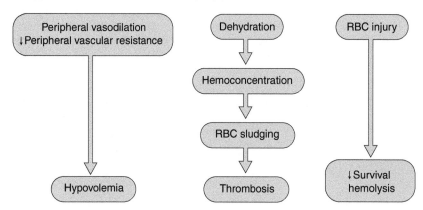

C Effect of Hyperthermia on the Hemostatic System

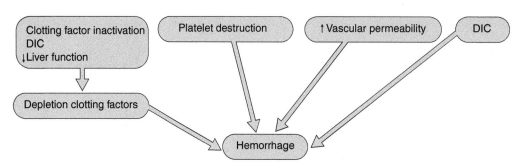

Diagnosis

Clinical signs can vary with the duration and severity of the hyperthermia. Increased rectal temperature and excessive panting are most obvious clinical signs (**Parts A, B,** and **C**). Panting is important since pyrexia caused by infection or inflammation will reset the hypothalamic thermoregulatory mechanism and panting will not be induced. Most animals present with injected mucous membranes, weakness, tachycardia, vomiting, and diarrhea. Body temperatures usually exceed 40.5°C (105°F). Stupor is an indication that the CNS has been affected. Convulsions or coma can follow in severely affected animals. The presence of cyanosis should alert the clinician to the presence of concurrent upper airway disease or secondary upper airway obstruction from laryngeal edema. Differential diagnosis for heatstroke should include infection, neoplasia, and toxicosis

Laboratory findings

The minimum database of the heat stroke patient consists of a complete blood count, a chemistry profile, and a urinalysis. Other useful tests include an arterial blood gas and a coagulation profile. Increases in hematocrit and total solids are due to hemoconcentration. Hypoxia stimulates the release of nucleated red blood cells from the bone marrow. Azotemia and proteinuria indicate the presence of acute renal damage. Hepatocellular necrosis and cholestasis lead to increases in liver enzymes including Alanine aminotransferase, serum alkaline phosphatase and total bilirubin. Elevated creatine phosphokinase and urine myoglobin suggest rhabdomyolysis. Electrolyte changes such as hypernatremia are due to dehydration. Initially, respiratory alkalosis from panting, as well as vomiting can lead to hypokalemia. Over time, hyperkalemia predominates with the development of acute renal failure, metabolic acidosis from lactic acid production, and rhabdomyolysis. A decreased platelet count with prolonged prothrombin time and partial thromboplastin times can occur with the development of DIC.

Management

Emergency measures to normalize the body temperature must be initiated as soon as heat stroke is suspected. In human heat stroke patients, survival has been linked to the time until normalization of body temperature. Owners should be instructed to begin the cooling process before bringing their pet to the hospital. The use of hoses, cold water baths, wet towels, and fans can help with rapid cooling. Other cooling measures include cold water enemas and intravenous fluids with the lines cooled in an ice bath. The use of ice baths is discouraged as this can lead to peripheral vasoconstriction which impairs heat dissipation, and also shivering which can increase heat production. Cooling measures should be stopped at 39.5°C (103°F) to avoid hypothermia since temperatures continue to fall after cooling measures have been discontinued.

After cooling measures have been initiated, goals of therapy involve volume replacement, stabilization of cell membranes, and protection against infection. Fluid therapy is crucial as extreme dehydration is present. In addition, decreased cardiac output causes decreased effective circulating volume and consequently hypovolemia. Isotonic solutions such as 0.9% NaCl or lactated Ringers should be initiated at a shock dose of 90 ml/kg/hr, and continued based on the cardiovascular and hemodynamic state of the patient.

Broad-spectrum antibiotic therapy should be initiated immediately, as the heat stroke patient is predisposed to infection and sepsis. Bacterial translocation occurs as the integrity of the intestinal mucosa becomes compromised, and decreased activity of the hepatic reticuloendothelial system also leads to general immunosuppression.

Corticosteroid therapy can be used to decrease cerebral edema especially if signs of central nervous system disturbances are present (dexamethasone sodium phosphate 1 mg/kg IV or prednisolone sodium succinate 5–11 mg/kg IV). Mannitol should be avoided initially to avoid circulatory collapse of the cardiovascularly compromised patient.

Acepromazine (0.05-1 mg/kg IV) or diazepam (1 mg/kg IV) can be used if severe shivering occurs. Diazepam should also be used as needed for seizures. The alpha blocking effects of acepromazine can also help counteract peripheral vasoconstriction associated with aggressive cooling measures. Hypotension associated with acepromazine use can be avoided with concurrent fluid therapy.

The use of antipyretics should be avoided as the hyperthermia of heat stroke patients is not caused by resetting of the hypothalamic temperature regulating mechanism. Nonsteroidal anti-inflammatory drugs should also be avoided due to the risk of causing GI bleeding, disturbed platelet function, and impaired renal function.

If cyanosis, increased respiratory effort and stridor are present, concurrent upper airway disease or laryngeal edema secondary to excessive panting should be suspected, and an emergency tracheostomy may be needed. Anti-arrhythmic therapy with lidocaine may be required if cardiac ventricular arrhythmias are severe enough to compromise perfusion. If DIC is present, both heparin and blood products such as fresh frozen plasma or whole blood should be used a needed.

Prognosis for the heatstroke patient is guarded. If hyperthermia is corrected immediately, systemic thermal injury may be minimal and chances of recovery can be fair. The development of acute renal failure, stupor or coma, and DIC can indicate a grave prognosis.

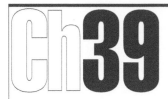

Hypothermia I: Pathophysiology

Armelle DeLaforcade and Nishi Dhupa

A   Predisposing Factors for Hypothermia

<u>Decreased heat production</u>
Neonates
Cachexia
Anesthesia
Cardiac disease
Immobility

<u>Increased heat loss</u>
Exposure (cold water, environmental)
Trauma
Surgery
Drugs-anesthetics (barbiturates, phenothiazines), ethylene glycol

<u>Disorders of thermoregulation</u>
Hypothyroidism
Adrenal insufficiency
CNS disorders (trauma, neoplasia, edema)

B   Treatment of Hypothermia

Minimize further heat loss (passive re-warming)
    Adequate for patients with mild hypothermia (>90°F)
    Dry the patient, protect from cold surfaces
    Blankets, towels
    Normothermia restored by intrinsic heat production mechanism (shivering)

Active external re-warming
    Hot water bottles
    Heating pads
    Heat lamps
    Heated incubators
    Intravenous fluids (to restore circulating blood volume)

Active core re-warming
    Warmed intravenous fluids
    Warmed humidified air by mask
    Warm peritoneal lavage
    Gastric or urinary bladder lavage
    Warm water enemas

Hypothermia is defined as a condition whereby core body temperature falls below physiologically normal levels. In veterinary medicine, hypothermia can be caused by prolonged exposure to a cold environment or can occur secondary to a disease process which alters thermoregulation (**Part A**). Hypothermia can also be induced with the use of certain drugs or anesthetic agents. The effect of hypothermia on the body systems depends on the severity and length of cold exposure. A high mortality rate can be associated with this condition. In animals, hypothermia is considered mild at temperatures ranging from 32°C–37°C (90°F–99°F), moderate at 28°C–32°C (82°F–90°F), and severe when below 28°C (82°F).

Physiology

Core body temperature is maintained through a homeostatic balance of heat loss and heat retention controlled by the thermoregulatory center in the hypothalamus. In response to a cold environment, both heat retention and heat production are initiated in an effort to maintain normal physiological temperature. Heat retention is mainly achieved by behavioral changes such as seeking warmth or huddling together, as well as reflex physiological changes such as piloerection (which traps a layer of warm air against the skin) and peripheral vasoconstriction. Increased cellular metabolic rate and involuntary motor activity (consisting mostly of shivering) are the principal means of heat generation. Failure of these mechanisms to restore normal core body temperatures lead to hypothermia.

Predisposing Factors

Predisposing factors for hypothermia are listed in **Part A**. Animals at risk for decreased heat production include neonates and cachexic animals due to decreased muscle, fat, and glycogen reserves. Certain disorders can also impair thermoregulation. Hypothyroidism decreases core body temperature by altering the hypothalamic setpoint and the shivering response. Adrenal insufficiency decreases the body's ability to respond to stress or cold, and central nervous system disorders can affect hypothalamic function. Anesthesia and surgery place animals at risk for the development of hypothermia. This occurs through immobility (decreased skeletal muscle activity), inhalation of nonhumidified anesthetic gases, and decreased metabolic rate. Surgical procedures further contribute to the development of hypothermia through exposure of open body cavities. Drugs such as ethylene glycol, barbiturates, and phenothiazines can cause peripheral vasodilation leading to increased heat loss, decreased shivering, and consequent hypothermia (**Part B**).

Pathophysiology

In response to mild hypothermia (90–99°F), increases in catecholamine release lead to peripheral vasoconstriction, shivering, and increases in heart rate, cardiac output, and blood pressure. This leads to decreased heat loss and increased endogenous heat production. These compensatory mechanisms begin to fail when hypothermia becomes more severe. At temperatures ranging from 82–90°F, heart rate and cardiac output begin to decline. The shivering response is decreased, muscles become rigid, and mental depression becomes apparent.

Electrocardiogram changes in response to hypothermia are due to decreased conduction and include lengthened P-R, QRS, and Q-T intervals as well as bradycardia. In humans, an 'Osborne' or 'J' wave represents an acute ST segment elevation that can be seen with temperatures between 90°F and 92°F (32–33°C). Although pathognomonic for severe hypothermia in humans, the Osborne wave has rarely been documented in small animals. At temperatures below 82°F (28°C), animals are predisposed to ventricular arrhythmias, ventricular tachycardia, and ventricular fibrillation that is unresponsive to mechanical defibrillation.

Central nervous system changes in response to hypothermia include depression followed by loss of consciousness. Cellular metabolism is decreased to such a degree that severely hypothermic animals are able to meet their metabolic demands in the presence of profound bradycardia and asystole. For this reason, severely hypothermic animals often appear dead.

Respiratory changes in response to hypothermia include initial tachypnea followed by decreased respiratory rate and tidal volume. Hypothermic patients are at risk for bronchopneumonia due to decreased mucociliary activity, the development of bronchiolar and alveolar edema, and subsequent atelectasis. Not only is oxygen diffusion across alveolar membranes reduced, but a shift in the oxygen-hemoglobin dissociation curve to the left in response to hypothermia leads to decreased dissociation of oxygen from oxyhemoglobin molecules and decreased oxygen delivery to tissues.

Renal changes in response to hypothermia contribute to a phenomenon called cold diuresis. Decreased antidiuretic hormone levels due to an increase in blood volume from the peripheral vasoconstriction seen initially in hypothermia leads to increased glomerular filtration rate (GFR). Increased GFR along with decreased tubular reabsorption and the presence of hyperglycemia leads to diuresis which can result in severe dehydration and azotemia. Although the liver is fairly resistant to damage induced by hypothermia, glycogen depletion and decreased metabolic function can occur.

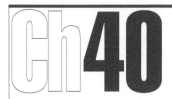

Hypothermia II: Diagnosis and Treatment

Armelle DeLaforcade and Nishi Dhupa

A   Predisposing Factors for Hypothermia

<u>Decreased heat production</u>
Neonates
Cachexia
Anesthesia
Cardiac disease
Immobility

<u>Increased heat loss</u>
Exposure (cold water, environmental)
Trauma
Surgery
Drugs-anesthetics (barbiturates, phenothiazines), ethylene glycol

<u>Disorders of thermoregulation</u>
Hypothyroidism
Adrenal insufficiency
CNS disorders (trauma, neoplasia, edema)

B   Treatment of Hypothermia

Minimize further heat loss (passive re-warming)
    Adequate for patients with mild hypothermia (>90°F)
    Dry the patient, protect from cold surfaces
    Blankets, towels
    Normothermia restored by intrinsic heat production mechanism (shivering)

Active external re-warming
    Hot water bottles
    Heating pads
    Heat lamps
    Heated incubators
    Intravenous fluids (to restore circulating blood volume)

Active core re-warming
    Warmed intravenous fluids
    Warmed humidified air by mask
    Warm peritoneal lavage
    Gastric or urinary bladder lavage
    Warm water enemas

Diagnosis

Diagnosis of hypothermia is based on history of exposure to cold. If known exposure to a cold environment is not evident, predisposing factors that can lead to hypothermia must be considered (**Part A**). Clinical signs of hypothermia vary with degree of severity. Mildly affected animals may show lethargy, mental depression, and shivering. Moderately affected animals may have lost the shivering reflex and may be stuporous, uncoordinated, or unconscious. Severely affected animals may be collapsed with fixed and dilated pupils and little or no respiratory and cardiac sounds. A minimum database should include a packed cell volume, total solids, blood glucose level, and an azostik. Further testing should include a complete blood count, chemistry profile, coagulation panel, a thyroid level, and a blood gas. Evaluation of true body temperature may be difficult since conventional thermometers do not read below 94°F (34.4°C).

Laboratory Findings

Lactic acidosis as a result of decreased oxygen exchange, shivering, and decreased peripheral tissue perfusion leads to the development of a metabolic acidosis in hypothermic animals. Mildly affected animals may have a mixed respiratory alkalosis and metabolic acidosis due to tachypnea.

Isotonic dehydration and splenic contraction in hypothermic animals results in increased hematocrit, hemoglobin, and total solids. Severe hemoconcentration can lead to increased blood viscosity which can contribute to neurological signs. Leukopenia and thrombocytopenia results from sequestration of white blood cells and platelets within the spleen and perivascular tissues. Progressive thrombocytopenia can also be due to disseminated intravascular coagulation (DIC) and activation of the clotting cascade as a result of prolonged hypoperfusion of extremities. In addition to low platelet numbers, functional abnormalities of both platelets and clotting factors occur secondary to hypothermia and are reversed with rewarming.

Low serum sodium (Na^+) and high serum potassium (K^+) can be seen due to depressed activity of sodium-potassium pumps in cell membranes. Although serum levels of Na^+ and K^+ may be altered, total body concentrations of Na^+ and K^+ are often normal. During the rewarming period, metabolic acidosis caused by poor peripheral perfusion can lead to further increases in K^+ levels due to the K^+/H^+ ion shift. Hyperglycemia and mild ketosis may develop as a result of stress-induced gluconeogenesis and both depressed insulin release from the pancreas and blocked action of insulin on receptor sites.

Treatment

An animal with profound hypothermia should be handled to avoid precipitating ventricular fibrillation. If this occurs shock defibrillation can be attempted but may not be effective until the rewarming process is initiated. In humans bretylium tosylate is used to augment electrical defibrillation. Anti-arrhythmic medication should not be used until body temperature exceeds 30°C (86°F). Repeated administrations should be avoided since they will accumulate and reach toxic levels when the patient is rewarmed.

Successful treatment of the severely hypothermic patient is based on support of vital organ systems, prevention of further heat loss, and restoration of body temperature to a normal range (**Part B**). Rewarming techniques are chosen based on the severity of hypothermia and include passive rewarming, active external rewarming, and active core rewarming. Passive rewarming involves the use of insulation materials such as blankets and allows the patients' intrinsic heat production mechanism (shivering) to correct the hypothermia. Passive rewarming is adequate for stable patients with mild hypothermia (>90°F). Active external rewarming techniques involve the use of exogenous heat sources (hot water bottles, heating pads, and heat lamps). Active rewarming can cause vasodilation, hypotension, and hypovolemic shock through a decrease in circulating blood volume. To prevent this phenomenon known as rewarming shock, heat should be applied only to the thorax leaving the extremities cool. This allows the body's core temperature to rise leaving the extremities to be perfused and warmed once the body is able to meet its metabolic demands. The administration of warmed crystalloid intravenous fluids is an essential component of active external rewarming as it leads to rapid restoration of effective circulating blood volume. Electric heating blankets should be avoided and radiant heat sources should be placed at least 29 inches from the patient to prevent burns. Active core rewarming is the most aggressive method of treating hypothermia and should be used in severe cases. In animals, warm peritoneal lavage is the best option. Stock dialysate solution can be used, or alternating lactated Ringer's solution and 5% dextrose in water. The dialysate should be warmed in a water bath to 45°C (113°F). A total of 50 ml/kg/exchange should be allowed to flow into the peritoneal cavity and then drained by gravity flow. Normothermia should be restored in 6–8 exchanges. Other possibilities include warm gastric or bladder lavage, airway rewarming (supplying warm humidified air by mask or tube), and warm water enemas. This type of rewarming allows rapid restoration of body temperature and avoids problems like shock encountered with active external rewarming.

In addition to rewarming techniques, supportive care is extremely important in managing the hypothermic patient. Continuous monitoring of body temperature should be performed, and all rewarming measures should be stopped at 96°F to prevent hyperthermia. The electrocardiogram should be closely monitored as should urine output. Use warmed intravenous fluids consisting of a balanced electrolyte solution. In severely hypothermic animals, lactated Ringer's solution should be avoided due to the compromised liver's inability to metabolize lactate. If the hypothermic patient is clinically bleeding but has a normal coagulation panel, this is likely due to functional factor abnormalities related to hypothermia that will resolve with rewarming. If the prothrombin and partial thromboplastin times are prolonged, fresh frozen plasma should be administered. Once normothermia has been restored, the patient should be continuously monitored for possible complications including pneumonia, acute respiratory distress syndrome, acute renal failure, and pancreatitis.

Ch41 Nosocomial Infections

Justine A. Johnson

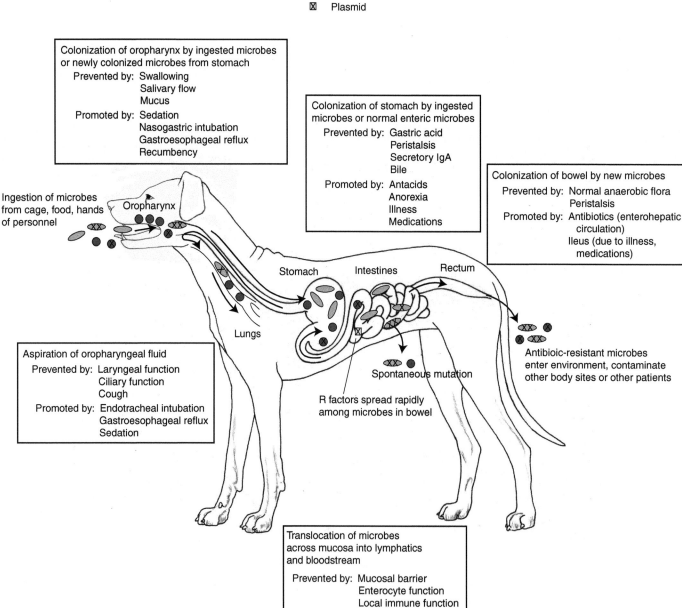

Normal gram positive flora

Normal gram negative or anaerobic flora

Gene carrying antibiotic resistance (R factors)

Plasmid

Colonization of oropharynx by ingested microbes
or newly colonized microbes from stomach
    Prevented by: Swallowing
                   Salivary flow
                   Mucus
    Promoted by: Sedation
                   Nasogastric intubation
                   Gastroesophageal reflux
                   Recumbency

Colonization of stomach by ingested
microbes or normal enteric microbes
    Prevented by: Gastric acid
                   Peristalsis
                   Secretory IgA
                   Bile
    Promoted by: Antacids
                   Anorexia
                   Illness
                   Medications

Colonization of bowel by new microbes
    Prevented by: Normal anaerobic flora
                   Peristalsis
    Promoted by: Antibiotics (enterohepatic
                   circulation)
                   Ileus (due to illness,
                   medications)

Ingestion of microbes
from cage, food, hands
of personnel

Oropharynx

Stomach   Intestines   Rectum

Lungs

Antibioic-resistant microbes
enter environment, contaminate
other body sites or other patients

Spontaneous mutation

Aspiration of oropharyngeal fluid
    Prevented by: Laryngeal function
                   Ciliary function
                   Cough
    Promoted by: Endotracheal intubation
                   Gastroesophageal reflux
                   Sedation

R factors spread rapidly
among microbes in bowel

Translocation of microbes
across mucosa into lymphatics
and bloodstream
    Prevented by: Mucosal barrier
                   Enterocyte function
                   Local immune function
    Promoted by: Medications
                   Enterocyte malnutrition
                   Illness/ debilitaton

Nosocomial infections are acquired during a patient's hospitalization. They are a cause of concern because they often occur in sick or debilitated patients, and because the organisms causing these infections are often resistant to commonly used antibiotics. The incidence of nosocomial infections in veterinary patients is increasing as a result of the increasing use of invasive devices and broad-spectrum antibiotics, which disrupt the body's natural defenses to bacterial infection. Bacteria associated with nosocomial infection may arise from normal endogenous populations on the patient's skin, oral cavity, or upper respiratory or GI tracts (**Figure**). It is not uncommon, however, for infections to arise due to inoculation with bacteria from the hospital environment that have developed antibiotic resistance. Nosocomial infections arising from any body site can lead to sepsis, organ failure, and death.

GI Tract

The stomach is typically a sterile environment because of the combined activities of salivary flow, mucus, secretory IgA, gastric acid, bile, and peristalsis. Bacteria gain access to the stomach by ingestion or retrograde flow from the intestines. Colonization of the stomach by these bacteria occurs if the acid level is altered by antacid medication, or if gastric function is affected by anorexia or ileus induced by medications or disease.

The lower intestine is inhabited mainly by anaerobic flora that prevent colonization of other bacterial populations. Antibiotics cause a decrease in the normal bacterial populations, allowing colonization by antibiotic-resistant organisms. Genes for antibiotic resistance occur randomly as a result of mutations, but also are transmitted rapidly among bacterial populations on plasmids. Bacteria may gain access to other body sites via translocation across the mucosa. This is most likely when there is mucosal disruption due to medications (e.g., steroids and NSAIDs), malnutrition of enterocytes (due to prolonged anorexia), or illness. Bacteria in the intestines also may be eliminated in the vomitus and feces of these patients, infecting other body sites or other patients.

Respiratory Tract

The lower respiratory tract is protected from bacterial colonization by normal laryngeal and ciliary function, coughing, and the immune system. These barriers are altered in recumbent and debilitated animals, especially when endotracheal tubes and mechanical ventilators are in use. The upper respiratory tract is normally inhabited by gram-positive organisms. These organisms may be introduced into the lower respiratory tract during endotracheal tube placement or may be aspirated around the endotracheal tube. Gastroesophageal reflux can lead to aspiration of oropharyngeal fluid containing gram-negative bacilli that have colonized the stomach.

Urinary Tract

Most nosocomial urinary tract infections occur secondary to the use of urinary catheters. Enteric organisms, usually from fecal contamination of the external portion of the catheter, are the most common bacteria isolated in urinary tract infections. The risk of urinary tract infection is increased with prolonged catheterization. If an indwelling catheter is placed, it should be connected to a closed collection system. Retrograde flow of the collected urine back into the bladder should be prevented, and the catheter site kept clean. Prophylactic antibiotic administration during catheterization may promote the development of antibiotic-resistant bacteria and should be avoided.

Bloodstream

Infections of the bloodstream can occur secondary to bacterial translocation across gut mucosa, wound infections, or infections at any body site. However, the most common source is infection at the site of IV catheters. The catheter may become contaminated by skin flora during insertion, by bacteria on the hands of hospital personnel, by contamination of IV fluids during manipulation of fluid lines, or rarely by blood-borne pathogens during existing bacteremia. Catheter infections are prevented by using an aseptic technique during catheter placement, protecting the catheter from soiling during use, and minimizing the opportunities for fluid contamination via injection ports and disconnected fluid lines.

Surgical Wounds

Infection of surgical wounds requires introduction of bacteria, but the amount of bacteria necessary to cause infection depends on the condition of the wound. The presence of hematomas, necrotic tissue, dead space, suture reaction, and altered circulation greatly increases the chance of wound infection. An aseptic technique should be used during surgical preparation and throughout the procedure. If drains are necessary, they should be covered or attached to a closed suction apparatus.

If the surgical site is known to be contaminated with bacteria, or if a hollow organ is to be opened during surgery, perioperative antibiotics should be administered. A broad-spectrum antibiotic is given 30 minutes prior to surgery and repeated every 2–3 hours during the procedure. Antibiotics are continued if known contamination of the surgery site occurred.

Prevention and Treatment

General strategies for the prevention of nosocomial infection involve strict adherence to hygiene. Hospital equipment and the hands of hospital personnel are common sources of nosocomial infections. Hand washing before handling each patient, and the use of disposable gloves can greatly reduce the incidence of microbe transmission. Careful aseptic technique should be used during the placement of IV and urinary catheters, as well as during preoperative surgical preparation and surgical procedures. Invasive devices pose a risk to the patient as long as they are in place, and should always be removed as soon as possible. Patients with suspected infections, especially those with diarrhea, should be isolated and handled by personnel wearing barrier clothing such as gloves and gowns. Weak, debilitated, and immunocompromised patients also should be handled by personnel with barrier clothing to prevent the introduction of new microbes.

Because antibiotic use promotes the development of hospital pathogens with antibiotic resistance, antibiotics should be used judiciously. Prophylactic antibiotics are rarely indicated. Antibiotics used in the treatment of infection should be selected based on the required spectrum of activity, as well as results of bacterial culture and antibiotic sensitivity testing.

It is important for hospital personnel to be aware of any patterns of infections, such as an increase in IV catheter infection rates, or the repeated appearance of specific microbial populations on bacterial cultures. It may be necessary to adopt and enforce specific hospital policies regarding staff hygiene, antibiotic use, and equipment disinfection.

Research is being conducted to improve the invasive devices that are associated with nosocomial infection in human patients. However, advances in technology are unlikely to be as effective as careful attention to hygiene in the prevention of nosocomial disease.

Ch42 Respiratory Distress

Daniel V. Hecht

A Causes of Dyspnea

Major Airway Obstruction

Collapsing trachea, hypoplastic trachea
Stenotic nares
Elongated soft palate
Eversion of the lateral ventricles
  of the larynx
Foreign body
Laryngeal paralysis
Trauma

Parenchymal Disease

Cardiogenic edema
Noncardiogenic edema
ARDS
Electrocution
Seizures
Smoke inhalation
Parasitic
Pneumonia
Pulmonary contusion

Pleural Space Disease

Chylothorax
Diaphragmatic hernia
Hemothorax
Neoplasia
Pneumothorax
Pyothorax
Transudate

Small Airway Obstruction

Asthma
Atelectasis
Trauma

Miscellaneous

Fractured ribs
Metabolic disease
Neuromuscular disease
Right-to-left cardiac shunt
Thromboembolic disease (PTE)

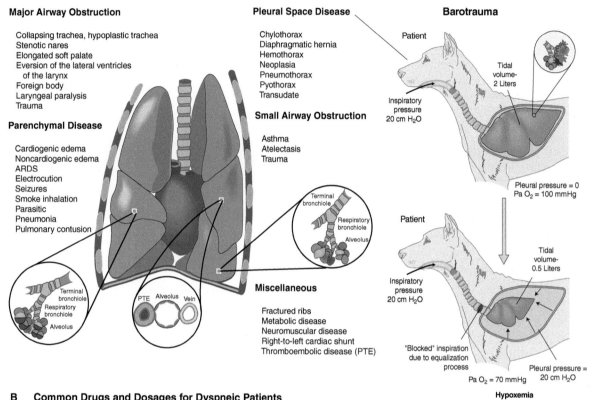

Barotrauma

Patient
Tidal volume- 2 Liters
Inspiratory pressure 20 cm H_2O
Pleural pressure = 0
Pa O_2 = 100 mmHg

Patient
Tidal volume- 0.5 Liters
Inspiratory pressure 20 cm H_2O
"Blocked" inspiration due to equalization process
Pa O_2 = 70 mmHg
Pleural pressure = 20 cm H_2O

Hypoxemia

Terminal bronchiole
Respiratory bronchiole
Alveolus

PTE Alveolus Vein

B Common Drugs and Dosages for Dyspneic Patients

Drug	Dose	Comments
Analgesics/sedatives		
Butorphanol tartate	Dogs: 0.1-0.8 mg/kg IV, IM, SQ every 4-8 hr prn	
	Cats: 0.1-0.2 mg/kg IV, IM, SQ every 4-6 hr prn	
Diazepam	Dogs: 5-15 mg/kg IV	
	Cats: 1.0-2.5 mg IV	
Medetomidine	10-20 µg/kg IM	Use caution with cardiac disease
Atipamezole	50 µg/kg IM	Medetomidine antagonist
Bronchodilators		
Aminophylline	Dogs: 6-11 mg/kg IV, PO every 8 hr	
	Cats: 4 mg/kg PO or slow IV every 12 hr	
Epinephrine	0.5 mL of 1:10,000 dilution IM, SQ	
Terbutaline	Dogs and cats: 0.01 mg/kg SQ every 4 hr or 1.25 mg PO per cat	
Corticosteroids		
Dexamethasone sodium phosphate	0.2-1.0 mg/kg IV, IM, SQ	
Prednisolone sodium succinate	5-10 mg/kg IV, IM	
Diuretics		
Furosemide	2-4 mg/kg IV, IM, every 2-12 hr	
Spironolactone	2-4 mg/kg PO every 12 hr	
Inotropes		
Digoxin	0.005-0.010 mg/kg PO every 12 hr	
Dobutamine hydrochloride	Dogs: 2.5-10.0 µg/kg/min IV	CRI
	Cats: 0.5-3.0 µg/kg/min IV	
Dopamine	3-10 µg/kg/min IV	CRI
Venodilators		
Nitroglycerin	1/8-1/2 inch topically every 6 hr	
Sodium nitroprusside	Dogs: 1-10 µg/kg/min IV	CRI

The goal in managing patients with respiratory distress is to optimize oxygen delivery to and carbon dioxide removal from the cells. There are 3 main determinants of the delivery of oxygen to the tissues: cardiac output, hemoglobin concentration, and the partial pressure of oxygen in the arterial system (PaO_2).

Pathophysiology

Hypoxemia (inadequate arterial oxygenation) is the condition where the PaO_2 is <60 mm Hg. There are 4 mechanisms by which hypoxemia occurs: hypoventilation, diffusion impairment, ventilation-perfusion mismatch, and intrapulmonary shunts. Hypoventilation can be caused by sedatives, muscle weakness, neurological disease, thoracic cage trauma, or upper-airway disease. There is always an increase in the partial pressure of carbon dioxide in the arterial system ($PaCo_2$) as well as a decrease in the PaO_2. Diffusion impairment occurs when the blood-gas barrier is thickened, which can occur with pneumonia or acute respiratory distress syndrome (ARDS). Oxygen absorption is decreased because of the greater distance it must travel to reach the capillaries. A ventilation-perfusion mismatch is an imbalance between pulmonary ventilation and capillary blood flow, commonly seen with chronic obstructive pulmonary disease (COPD), congestive heart failure, or pulmonary thromboembolism. A shunt occurs when blood reaches the right atrium without passing through ventilated areas of lung. Examples include intrapulmonary arterial-venous fistulas, right-to-left cardiac shunt, or a severely consolidated lung lobe (**Part A**).

Clinical Signs and Presentation

The clinical signs associated with hypoxemia are characterized by abnormalities in respiratory rate, effort, and character. The animal may demonstrate an abnormally wide stance (with extension of the head and neck), panting, cyanosis or pale mucous membranes, and orthopnea. Tachycardia, weakness, stridor, and coughing are commonly seen. Most animals in distress present with a sense of panic or air hunger, and the respiratory rate can be increased or decreased. Careful observation of the animal is important in localizing the lesion and should always be done before any manipulation or hands-on examination.

Diagnostics

A brief history is key to the initial diagnostic approach and can be taken as the examination is started. It is important to note whether there is increased respiratory effort on inspiration or expiration or both. Is the breathing noisy or quiet? Is it rapid and shallow or slow with increased effort? Cats in severe respiratory distress do not always exhibit clinical signs to the same degree as dogs. Cats can be extremely hypoxemic and yet only show tachypnea and mildly increased respiratory effort. Throughout the initial examination, it is critical to administer oxygen and occasionally a tranquilizer. Considerations for tranquilizers include drugs such as butorphanol (which has minimal respiratory and cardiac depression) or medetomidine (which is reversible with atipamezole). These approaches will help to make the examination and diagnostic procedures easier and less stressful.

It is important to choose initially the appropriate tests that will give the most information with the least stress. This is especially true with cats. Measurement of the saturation of hemoglobin with oxygen by pulse oximeter (SpO_2) is very useful and relatively nonstressful. However, SpO_2 may not always be measurable because of poor perfusion or movement by the animal. An arterial blood gas (ABG) analysis is the "gold standard" when evaluating a dyspneic patient, as it gives an accurate assessment of arterial oxygen, carbon dioxide, bicarbonate, and pH. Samples for ABG are sometimes difficult to obtain. Thoracocentesis can be therapeutic as well as diagnostic when a pneumothorax or pleural effusion is suspected. Thoracic radiographs can provide substantial information and as a general rule should be done as soon as the animal is stabilized. If the animal does not stabilize and is deteriorating, radiographs are also indicated. A minimum laboratory evaluation consisting of a complete blood cell count, biochemical profile, and urinalysis should be performed in all cases. Heartworm testing is recommended in any dog or cat with respiratory distress and evidence of right-sided heart disease, pulmonary artery enlargement, or possible allergic lung disease. Fecal flotation and Baermann sedimentation tests will help detect parasitic pneumonitis caused by *Aelurostrongylus*, Filaroides, and *Paragonimus* spp. Indications for a transtracheal aspiration and broncho-alveolar lavage to provide samples for microbiological culture and cytological evaluation include all causes of lower-airway disease and noncardiogenic intrapulmonary disease.

A presumptive diagnosis of congestive heart failure (CHF) can be made based on a prominent heart murmur, crackles, a hilar interstitial pattern on thoracic radiographs, or coughing up of pink foamy fluid.

Treatment

Oxygen is good; use it. It is quick and easy to administer. The easiest method for oxygen administration is the flow-by technique, where an oxygen line is held near the animal's face and oxygen is flowing at a rate of 5–10 L/min. Other simple effective ways to administer oxygen are via face mask, into an E-collar apparatus with plastic wrap covering 90% of the front opening, or into a large clear plastic bag placed over the animal's head. With these last two techniques, an oxygen line is inserted into the temporary tent area; this allows the clinician to perform ongoing examinations. An oxygen cage provides a fast effective source for oxygen administration, but limits hands-on examination. For animals presenting in concurrent shock, this condition should be addressed immediately after oxygen administration is initiated. Following resuscitation from shock, judicious use of fluids is indicated should there be subsequent evidence that pulmonary edema or severe pulmonary contusions are present.

Many cats present with dyspnea and have findings on thoracic radiographs that can make it hard to differentiate CHF, asthma, and pneumonia. In these cases, treatment sometimes needs to be broad based, consisting of administration of bronchodilators, diuretics, and antibiotics as well as oxygen (**Part B**). Terbutaline can be given by injection or aerosol for a more direct effect. Occasionally a short-acting corticosteroid such as dexamethasone sodium phosphate is used to counteract the allergic response associated with feline asthma. Echocardiograms and transtracheal washes may be needed with these patients to determine a definitive diagnosis and tailor the long-term treatment protocol to the specific disease.

Most dyspneic animals need aggressive treatment before a definitive diagnosis is made. In general, diuretics are only effective for treatment of cardiogenic pulmonary edema, as there is no conclusive evidence that there is any benefit to use these drugs in animals with noncardiogenic pulmonary edema or pulmonary contusions. CHF is treated with positive inotropes such as digoxin, Dobutamine, or dopamine, a venodilator such as nitroglycerin or nitroprusside, and diuretics (see **Part B**). Both dopamine and nitroprusside must be administered carefully as a constant-rate infusion, and blood pressure must be monitored closely.

Finally, when other modes of treatment are insufficient to prevent hypoxemia, a ventilator should be considered. Ventilation therapy is reserved for patients that do not respond to supplemental oxygen therapy and medications.

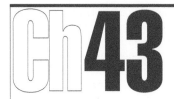

Seizures I: Pathophysiology

Theresa O'Toole

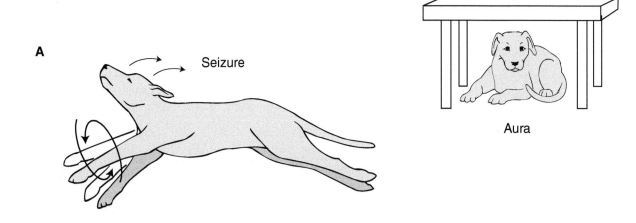

A

Seizure

Aura

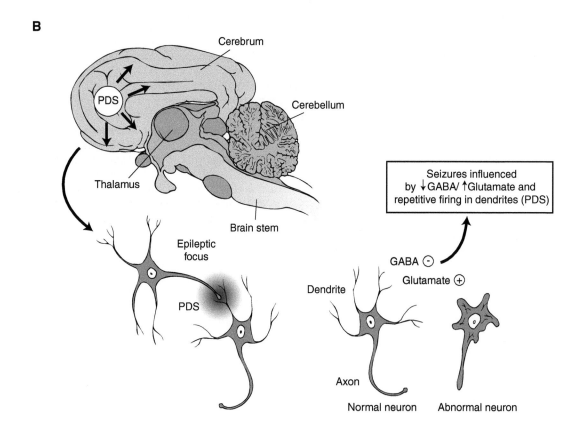

B

Cerebrum

Cerebellum

PDS

Thalamus

Brain stem

Epileptic focus

PDS

Dendrite

GABA ⊖

Glutamate ⊕

Axon

Normal neuron   Abnormal neuron

Seizures influenced
by ↓GABA/↑Glutamate and
repetitive firing in dendrites (PDS)

The CNS consists of a vast array of circuits of neurons functioning to produce excitatory and inhibitory neurotransmission. A seizure results when neurons or populations of neurons aberrantly synchronize to produce repetitive burst firing, causing a transient alteration in behavior. Epilepsy, which is a syndrome of CNS dysfunction, is characterized by recurrent and unpredictable seizures. Many types of seizures, conventionally regarded as resulting from an imbalance in neuronal excitatory and inhibitory interactions, are recognized.

Categorization

Seizures are broadly characterized on the basis of their origins: generalized or partial. In addition, several subtypes of seizures are described within each of these 2 categories. A partial seizure arises from part of a cerebral hemisphere and is thought to be the result of a focal brain lesion. A generalized seizure, alternatively, arises over both hemispheres simultaneously. A partial seizure can generalize secondarily. When a partial seizure precedes a generalized seizure, it is referred to as an *aura* (**Part A**).

The generalized seizure usually is characterized by involuntary, clinically symmetrical, physical movements and loss of consciousness. These movements are typically described as clonic (repetitive muscle contraction and relaxation), tonic (muscle contraction), myoclonic (rhythmic clonic), or any combination of these signs. Historically referred to as grand mal, this is the typical convulsive motor seizure. Alternatively, a generalized seizure may be mild, characterized, for example, by bilaterally fine facial twitches. Absence seizures (petit mal) are generalized seizures as well, but differ from the characteristic convulsive motor seizure in their clinical appearance and pathogenesis. A blank stare is typical of the absence seizure. The seizure (ictal period) may be preceded by an aura in the preictal period, during which the animal may appear restless or hide, and is usually followed by a postictal period, during which disorientation, exhaustion, or transient neurological signs such as loss of menace or circling may be observed.

Partial seizures are broadly classified as simple or complex and are characterized by asymmetrical clinical signs. Simple partial seizures involve no loss of consciousness, whereas complex partial seizures are characterized by altered mental states. Complex partial seizures include temporal and frontal lobe epilepsies, as well as those historically described as psychomotor seizures (stereotypical behavior such as tail chasing).

Physiology

CNS function is derived by the action of excitatory and inhibitory neurotransmission (**Part B**). The primary excitatory neurotransmitter in the CNS is glutamate, and when binding to 1 of 3 glutamate receptors (NMDA, KA, AMPA) on the postsynaptic membrane, it causes depolarization of the nerve cell. Neurons implicated in epilepsy typically are arranged in layers in the cerebral cortex, receiving their initiating impulses from neurons located in the thalamic cortex. Impulses are sensed by receptors on the dendritic region of the neuron, and an action potential, or excitatory postsynaptic potential (EPSP), is generated at the axon hillock and transmitted down the axon to effect its purpose.

The resting membrane potential of a cell is maintained primarily by the selective permeability of ligand (ion)-gated and voltage-gated channels. The energy-dependent Na^+, K^+-AtPase pumps have an integral role in the maintenance of concentrations of extracellular sodium and intracellular potassium. A wave of depolarization is created if a change in membrane permeability allows an influx of sodium or calcium. When glutamate is released from the presynaptic membrane, it binds to its receptors postsynaptically and acts to open these selective sodium and calcium channels. When the cell is depolarized to its threshold, an EPSP is propagated at the axon region.

The predominant inhibitory neurotransmitter in the CNS is γ-aminobutyric acid (GABA). GABA is released from presynaptic membranes and acts on postsynaptic receptors to produce an inhibitory postsynaptic potential (IPSP). Cells are hyperpolarized when GABA receptors are bound by 1 of 2 mechanisms. If GABA A-type receptors are engaged, associated selectively permeable chloride channels open to allow an inward flux of negatively charged chloride; if GABA B-type receptors are bound, the outward flux of positively charged potassium is increased.

Pathophysiology

A paroxysmal depolarization shift (PDS) is a prolonged, exaggerated depolarization observed in the interictal state. Thought to originate in the dendritic zone, generation of the PDS requires afferent, excitatory input and recurrent and synchronous activity. The PDS is followed by a hyperpolarization phase, which is activated by outward potassium currents and feedback inhibition. Interference with these mechanisms results in disruption of the postdepolarization hyperpolarization phase, resulting in repetitive neuronal depolarization.

Traditionally thought of as hyperexcitable events, conditions that predispose to seizures have been presumed to involve an imbalance in neuronal excitatory and inhibitory influences. However, seizures most likely occur as a result of an upset in the balance of intricately complicated neuronal interactions. Transition to the ictal state occurs with the simultaneous breakdown of inhibitory systems while epileptogenic neurons are firing synchronously.

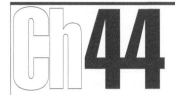

Seizures II: Diagnosis and Treatment

Therese O'Toole

A Common Causes of Seizures in Dogs
Structural Disease (SES)

1. Developmental (hydrocephalus, storage diseases)
2. Neoplasia (tumors most often associated with seizures are primary tumors of the frontal, olfactory, and parietal lobes; also nasal adenocarcinomas extending into the olfactory lobes)
3. Inflammatory
   a. Viral-canine, distemper, rabies
   b. Fungal-Cryptococcus neoformans, coccidioidomycosis
   c. Protozoal-toxoplasmosis, neospora
   d. Ricksettial-Rocky Mountain Spotted Fever, Ehrlichiosis
   e. Possibly immune mediated-granulomatous meningoencephalitis, necrotizing encephalitis (pugs, Maltese, and Yorkshire terriers)
   f. Brain abscess
4. Trauma
5. Cerebral vascular accident (coagulopathies, thrombocytopenia/thrombocytopathia)

Reactive Disease (RES)
1. Hepatic disease (hepatoencephalopathy)
2. Endocrine disease (hypothyroid)
3. Extrahepatic portal caval systemic shunts
4. Uremia
5. Hypertension
6. Hypoglycemia (insulin overdose, insulin-likeÐsecreting neoplasms)
7. Electrolyte abnormalities
   a. Sodium and serum osmolality shifts
   b. Hypercalcemia, hypocalcemia, hypomagnesemia, metabolic alkalosis
8. Hypoxemia (energy failure)
9. Congenital (disorders of oxidative phosphorylation)

Primary (PES)
1. Idiopathic epilepsy
   a. Common breeds: beagles, dachsunds, German shepherds, Keeshonds, Belgian shepherds, cocker spaniels, collies, golden retrievers, Irish setters, Labrador retrievers, miniature Schnauzers, poodles, Saint Bernards, Siberian Huskies, wire haired fox terriers

B Common Causes of Seizures in Cats
Structural Disease (SES)

1. Neoplasia (meningioma most common)
2. Inflammatory
   a. Fungal-Crytococcus neoformans infection
   b. Protozoal-Toxoplasmosis
   c. Brain abscess
   d. Viral-FIP
3. Feline ischemic encephalopathy
4. Primary nonsuppurative meningioencephalitis (unknown etiology, usually self-limiting)
5. Trauma
6. Cerebral vascular accident
   a. Coagulopathies
   b. Hypertension

Reactive Disease (RES)
1. Hepatic disease (hepatoencephalopathy)
2. Extrahepatic portal caval systemic shunts
3. Hypoglycemia (insulin overdose)
4. Polycythemia
5. Uremia
6. Hyperternsion
7. Electrolyte abnormalities
   a. Serum sodium and osmolality shifts
   b. Hypercalcemia, hypocalcemia, hypomagnesemia, metabolic alkalosis
8. Hypoxemia (energy failure)
9. Congenital (disorders of oxidative phosphorylation)
10. Hyperthyroidism

Primary (PES)
1. Idiopathic epilepsy (uncommon)

C Common Toxic Causes of Seizures

Increase Excitation of Neurons
1. Agents that inhibit sodium channel inactivation, prolonging the opening of sodium channels and thus cause repeated action potentials
   a. Pyrethrins/pyrethroids
   b. Plants (rhododendrons)
   c. Spider and scorpion toxins
   d. Type II pyrethrins (these also block GABA)
   e. Chlorinated hydrocarbons (insecticides-lindane, methoxyclor; these also prolong action potentials by disrupting potassium channels and decreasing hyperpolarization
2. Agents that increase glutaminergic tone
   a. Toxins found in some cycads, mushrooms and algae
3. Agents that increase calcium flux into neurons (phosphodiesterase inhibitors)
   a. Methylxanthines [theophylline, aminophylline, theobromine, (chocolate)]
4. Agents that increase acetylcholine levels
   a. Cholinesterase inhibitors (organophosphate, carbmate)

Decrease Inhibition of Neurons
1. Agents that interfere with GABA neurotransmission
   a. Biculine (found in bleeding heart and the wildflower Dutchman's-breeches)
   b. Cyclodience-organochlorine insecticides (eg. chlordane)
   c. Tremerogenic mycotoxins-Penitrem A-moldy foods, walnuts, cream cheese
   d. Metaldehyde-slug bait
2. Agents that interfere with glycine
   a. Strychnine

Interfere with Energy Metabolism
1. Agents that disrupt oxidative phosphorylation: bromethalin, hexachlorophene, rotenone, cyanide
2. Agents that decrease cofactors for tricarboxylic cycle: thiaminase-containing plants and fish
3. Agents that block delivery of necessary substrates for aerobic metabolism: carbon monoxide

Miscellaneous
1. Lead
2. Hydrocarbons: ethylene glycol, DEET, methanol, toluene, phenols, pine oils
3. Drugs: amphetamines, antibiotics (penicillin, cephalosporins), lidocaine, phenothiazines, antihistamines

Seizures in Small Animals

Seizures are a common presenting complaint in small-animal medicine, and it is useful to classify them broadly according to underlying precipitating causes. Secondary epileptic seizures (SESs) are seizures for which an identifiable structural brain lesion (e.g., developmental anomaly, neoplasia) can be determined. Reactive epileptic seizures (RESs) are those caused by extracranial problems (e.g., metabolic, systemic, or toxic insults). Those seizures for which a diagnostic work-up has identified no obvious structural or extracranial disease are classified as primary epileptic seizures (PESs).

Seizures in Dogs

According to retrospective studies, dogs presenting with recent-onset seizures are as likely to be diagnosed with structural brain disease (SESs) as they are to have no identifiable cause (PESs). A smaller number will have a toxic or metabolic/systemic cause. Dogs that have their first seizures at ages <1 year or >5 years are most likely to have SESs (e.g., developmental, neoplasia), and dogs that have their first seizures at ages 1–5 years are most likely to have PESs. In addition, PESs are more likely if recurrent seizures occur over a period >4 weeks; dogs with SESs are more likely to have recurrent seizures within a 4-week period, as are dogs with RESs. Dogs with SESs, moreover, may have normal initial findings on neurological examination; in 1 retrospective study, 75% of dogs with rostral cerebral tumors had normal interictal neurological findings (**Part A**).

Seizures in Cats

Complex partial seizures may represent the most common form of epilepsy in cats. Turning of the head, ventral flexion, or arching of the neck, frantic running or jumping, chewing, or "hallucinating" can be commonly seen. Generalized seizures may be recognized as typical, convulsive, tonic-clonic episodes; alternatively, generalized seizures may be mild, with the simple observation of bilateral pupil dilation or facial twitching. Some cats will have both partial and generalized seizures.

Primary epilepsy is uncommon in the cat. Most feline seizures result from structural brain disease or an extracranial problem. Moreover, cats more commonly show evidence of abnormalities on neurological examination. Probably the most common cause of seizures in cats is a primary, nonsuppurative meningoencephalitis of unknown etiology (possibly viral, usually self-limiting). Causes of reactive seizures are similar to those of canine reactive seizures, with the addition of polycythemia and hyperthyroidism (**Part B**).

Toxic Causes

Although seizures are a common clinical sign with exposure to many toxins or substances, it should be appreciated that toxic insults are an infrequent cause of seizures in animals. Toxins typically mediate their effects by either increasing excitatory (glutaminergic or cholinergic) or decreasing inhibitory (GABAergic or glycine) neurotransmission. In addition, they can directly interfere with the cell's ability to maintain resting membrane potential below threshold, or interfere with energy metabolism (decreased ATP levels hinder the function of the Na^+, K^+-ATPase pumps) by affecting the substrates for aerobic metabolism or oxidative phosphorylation (**Part C**).

Broad Categories of Antiepileptic Drugs (AEDs)

1. Drugs that increase inhibition by increasing seizure threshold (hyperpolarization).
   a. Barbiturates (phenobarbital, pentobarbital) and benzodiazepines act at the GABA receptor.
   b. Potassium (or sodium) bromide floods the chloride channel.
   c. Gabapentin is thought to facilitate presynaptic GABA release.
2. Drugs that decrease excitatory neurotransmission—felbamate, phenytoin, carbamazepine.
3. Modulators of membrane cation conductance such as ethosuximide, which reduces low-threshold, transient, voltage-dependent calcium conductance in thalamic neurons (used in treatment for absence seizures).

First Choices for AEDs

1. Emergency seizure control: IV medications.
   a. Diazepam is lipid soluble and crosses the blood-brain barrier to reach a therapeutic level within 10 minutes.
   b. Barbiturates: Use phenobarbital first. If seizures persist, then try pentobarbital. Try IV bolus first, followed by constant-rate infusion if seizures persist (consider intubation to maintain airway).
   c. Supportive care includes administration of thiamine, supplemental oxygen therapy, and IV dextrose if indicated.
2. Long-term seizure control: oral medications.
   a. Phenobarbital induces the cytochrome p_{450} system, so normal liver function is required for metabolism.
   b. Potassium bromide.
   c. Valium is given per rectum for emergency therapy at home.

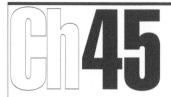

Intracranial Hypertension I: Causes and Consequences

Jeffrey Proulx

A Evaluation of the Brain-Injured Patient

Level of Consciousness
Cerebral or RAS lesion

Alert	Normal behavior and interactive
Depressed	Decreased responsiveness
Stuporous	Responds only to strong and painful stimuli
Comatose	Unresponsive

Cranial Nerve Exam
Pupillary light reflex (rule out ocular injury)

Intracranial lesion:

Unilateral mydriasis	Ipsilateral CN3 loss or midbrain lesion
Bilateral miosis	Severe midbrain lesion
Bilateral mydriasis	Severe advanced brain stem lesion
Unresponsive	Severe and extensive brain stem lesion
Oculocephalic reflex	
Present	Normal function of CN3, 4, 6, MLF, and CN8
Absent	Damage to CN3, 4, 6 or 8, or MLF (midbrain to medulla)
Strabismus	CN3, 4, 6 or midbrain to rostral medulla (3, 4, 6 nuclei)
Abnormal nystagmus/ head tilt	CN8 lesion peripheral or central, cerebellar, or brain stem lesion
Loss of facial sensation	CN5 lesion peripheral or central
Loss of facial motor	CN7 lesion peripheral or central lesion

Respiratory Patterns (rule out extracranial causes)

Cheyne-Stokes	Rostral brain stem lesion
Hyperventilation	Caudal mid-brain and pons lesion
Apneustic breathing	Caudal brain stem lesion

Motor (rule out extracranial causes)

Circling	Small circles-ipsilateral brain stem lesion
	Large circles-contralateral cerebral lesion
	Cerebellar and medulla lesion

Ataxia

Hemiparesis	Ipsilateral brain stem or contralateral cerebrum lesion
Spastic quadriparesis	Severe brain stem or diffuse cerebral lesion

Posture

Decerebrate rigidity	Severe midbrain pontine lesion
Decerebellate rigidity	Cerebellar lesion

CN= cranial nerve
MLF= Medial longitudinal fasciculus
RAS= Reticular Activating System

B Herniation

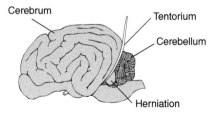

Cerebrum
Tentorium
Cerebellum
Herniation

C

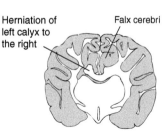

Herniation of left calyx to the right
Falx cerebri

D

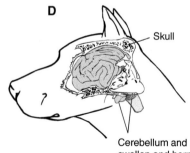

Skull

Cerebellum and medulla swollen and herniating out of foramen magnum

Elevated intracranial pressure (ICP) is a serious disorder in veterinary patients that if left untreated, can lead to permanent neurologic dysfunction, coma, and death. Many types of injuries and illnesses can lead to increased ICP. These include head trauma, cerebral tumors, infection, hemorrhage, and all causes of cerebral edema. Treatment of veterinary patients with elevated ICP needs to be directed at the primary disease as well as the intracranial hypertension itself (**Part A**).

Determinants of ICP

The balance between the enclosing rigid skull and the normal intracranial structures determines the ICP. These structures include brain tissue, CSF, and cerebral blood volume (CBV). With intracranial disease, additional pathological compartments may be present and can include interstitial edema, hemorrhage or hematoma, abscess, tumor, or an enlarged ventricular space. All components have the potential to expand and lead to increases in ICP.

Based on the Monro-Kellie doctrine, if expansion of 1 compartment occurs, normal ICP can only be preserved if a reciprocal compensation occurs in another compartment (intracranial compliance). Both the CSF and cerebral blood compartment are the major volume-buffering compartments, as brain tissue is relatively incompressible. ICP rises at the point at which no accommodation can occur. In general, rapid expansion of 1 compartment is not as easily accommodated in comparison to slower processes.

In acute intracranial hypertension, the CSF may be displaced to the spinal subarachnoid space or undergo hastened reabsorption, while with slower or chronic ICP elevation, CSF production may actually be reduced. CBV will be reduced based on its direct relationship with cerebral perfusion pressure (CPP). By definition, CPP is reduced with elevations in ICP, as shown by the equation CPP = Mean arterial pressure (MAP) −ICP, where the main driving force for blood flow to the brain (MAP) is lowered by the limitation of flow into the brain (ICP). Lowered CPP limits cerebral blood flow and consequently CBV.

Once intracranial compliance or buffering is exhausted, further increases in intracranial volume will result in exponential rises in ICP. This circumstance is exacerbated further when buffering compartments become converted to sources of increased intracranial compression. For instance, ventricular obstruction can lead to inadequate CSF drainage and an enlarged CSF space and further elevation in ICP.

Causes of Intracranial Hypertension

Intracranial pressure can be elevated with expansion of any of the 3 intracranial compartments: brain tissue (neurons, supporting cells, and interstitium), vascular space (arteries, microcirculation, and veins/sinuses), and CSF space. Primary or metastatic tumors with slow growth may be compensated initially by a reduction of mass within other structures, but eventually may increase the ICP by expansion alone, by obstructing CSF drainage, or by associated inflammation and bleeding. Localized bleeding (subdural, parenchymal, or subarachnoid hemorrhage) from trauma or coagulopathy, or abscesses have similar effects, with acute processes causing more rapid and severe elevations in ICP. Systemic or localized processes that cause diffuse inflammation (vasculitis, edema from seizure, trauma, hypoxemia and ischemia, reperfusion injury, disseminated intravascular coagulation, etc.) also will result in interstitial edema, expansion of brain tissue, and elevations in ICP.

Although most causes of intracranial hypertension lead to a decrease in cerebral blood flow, an increase in blood flow itself may instigate increased ICP by increasing CBV. For example, hypoventilation leads to an increase in carbon dioxide tension and secondary dilation of cerebral blood vessels, thereby raising ICP.

Consequences of Intracranial Hypertension

Herniation

With expansion of a particular compartment within the skull, herniation of the brain parenchyma is often a fatal consequence. Types of herniation include transtentorial (uncal) with increased pressure exerted on the brain stem **Part B**, subfalcine with herniation along the falx cerebri, (**Part C**), and foramen magnum herniation by caudal protrusion of the cerebellum and pressure exerted on the medulla oblongata (**Part D**). With disruption of the cerebral vascular supply and neural pathways within the brain stem (cardiorespiratory centers), coma and death typically result.

Cerebral Ischemic Response

Increases in ICP cause a reduction in cerebral perfusion (see earlier equation), relative ischemia, local acidosis, and an elevation in carbon dioxide. A direct sympathetic response originates from the brain stem and leads to an elevated heart rate and intense systemic arterial vasoconstriction in order to maintain adequate cerebral blood flow. Baroreceptors present in the aortic arch and carotid bodies may incite a reflexive slowing of the heart rate (Cushing's reflex). Therefore, the constellation of systemic hypertension and bradycardia should prompt an evaluation for CNS disease.

Intracranial Hypertension II: Treatment

Jeffrey Proulx

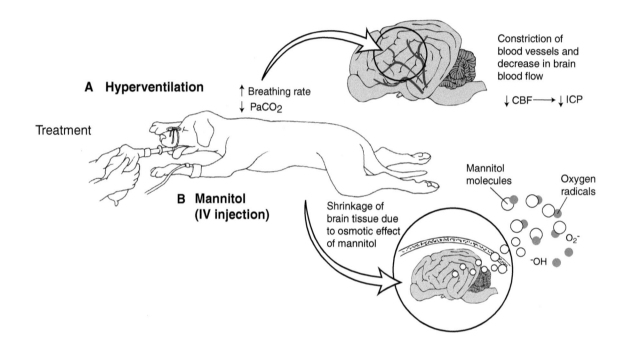

A Hyperventilation

↑ Breathing rate
↓ PaCO₂

Constriction of blood vessels and decrease in brain blood flow

↓ CBF ⟶ ↓ ICP

Treatment

B Mannitol (IV injection)

Shrinkage of brain tissue due to osmotic effect of mannitol

Mannitol molecules

Oxygen radicals

O₂⁻

⁻OH

Treatment of Intracranial Hypertension

Because there are many causes of intracranial hypertension, each potential treatment modality must be evaluated in regards to the specific disease and individual characteristics of the patient being treated. The general principles of treatment include efforts to treat the primary disease, maintenance of cerebral blood flow and oxygenation, and reduction of increased ICP. Care must be exercised in using treatment strategies that may decrease the ICP at the expense of cerebral blood flow. Any limitation to cerebral blood flow in a patient with intracranial disease may predispose to further secondary injury due to ischemia.

Head Elevation

Elevation of the head may decrease ICP by augmenting venous drainage and return to the systemic circulation. An adverse consequence is the potential to diminish arterial cerebral blood flow to an extent that may cause hypoxia. The current recommendation is for head positioning between 0 and 30 degrees. Additionally, it is probably more important to not perform any procedure that will compromise jugular venous return.

Hyperventilation

(**Part A**) Hyperventilation was at one time the mainstay of treating intracranial hypertension. Carbon dioxide directly alters cerebral blood vessel size (increasing carbon dioxide will dilate cerebral blood vessels and decreasing carbon dioxide constricts blood vessels) and therefore affects total CBV. The potential adverse consequence of hyperventilation (decreased carbon dioxide) is decreased regional or global cerebral blood flow. Although the ICP will be lowered, cerebral hypoxia or ischemia may result, thereby furthering brain injury. Patient management should include controlled ventilation to maintain adequate systemic oxygenation and maintain carbon dioxide pressure at approximately 30–35 mm Hg (normal is 40 ± 4 mm Hg).

Diuretics

Diuretics decrease ICP through 2 mechanisms. These include a reduction in the production of CSF (minimal) and a reduction in cerebral interstitial fluid volume by diuresis and dehydration. Diuretics such as furosemide are no longer recommended for most causes of increased ICP, as dehydration can set the stage for further brain injury as a result of dehydration, hypovolemia, and poor cerebral blood flow.

Oxygen and Mechanical Ventilation

Maintenance of oxygen delivery is essential to protecting brain tissue during episodes of intracranial hypertension. Maintenance of a normal red cell count, arterial oxygen tension, blood pressure, and appropriate ventilatory function will ensure maximization of cerebral oxygen delivery.

Mannitol

Mannitol is a hypertonic crystalloid that is very effective at decreasing ICP (**Part B**). Acting as an osmotic agent, mannitol will draw fluid from the cerebral interstitium (either normal or edematous interstitium), effectively augmenting cerebral compliance. It is especially useful in decreasing interstitial volume when cerebral edema is present. Other potential beneficial effects include oxygen free radical scavenging and reduced blood viscosity. The diuretic effect of mannitol must be combated to prevent dehydration and hypovolemia.

Hypertonic Saline

Hypertonic saline is a hyperosmotic crystalloid solution that acts similar to mannitol in drawing free water from the interstitium. An additional benefit includes a transient expansion of the intravascular volume, thereby supporting arterial blood pressure and cerebral perfusion.

Colloids

Synthetic colloids are high-molecular-weight substances with oncotic activity. Acting similar to mannitol and hypertonic saline solution, free water is drawn from the cerebral interstitium, and intravascular volume is expanded. The effects of synthetic colloids are much longer lived than the hypertonic crystalloids.

Corticosteroids

Although controversial, corticosteroids may be useful in diminishing interstitial edema associated with certain types of brain injury or mass lesions such as tumors, abscesses, or hemorrhage. Potential side effects of corticosteroids include GI hemorrhage, poor wound healing, and sodium and water retention, among others.

Barbiturates and Hypothermia

Both barbiturates and hypothermia will decrease the metabolic demand of cerebral tissue. If normal control of cerebral blood flow is intact, then a reduction in metabolic demand will cause an appropriate reduction in cerebral blood flow and volume. This will effect decreases in ICP without compromising adequate cerebral perfusion. Both treatments demand an increase in patient monitoring, as both treatments can precipitate hypotension and hypoventilation and cause decreased cerebral oxygen delivery.

CSF Aspiration

CSF aspiration is a treatment modality commonly used in human medicine to decrease the ICP. ICP is lowered by CSF aspiration through specially placed intracranial catheters. Intracranial catheters also allow the continuous monitoring of ICP and accurate titration of ICP-lowering therapy. The risks of CSF aspiration include herniation if only 1 particular compartment is decompressed relative to another structure separated by a rigid structure (e.g., tentorium). For this reason, patients with an ICP elevated >30 mm Hg are not considered candidates for CSF aspiration.

Craniotomy

Patients with extreme elevations of ICP, patients nonresponsive to other methods of ICP control, or patients with surgically accessible mass lesions (tumor, subdural hematoma) may benefit from surgical treatment. Lateral rostrotentorial craniotomy and duratomy are performed to directly decompress brain tissue.

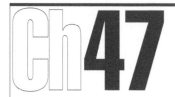

Acute Intrinsic Renal Failure I: Etiology and Pathophysiology

Robert J. Murtaugh

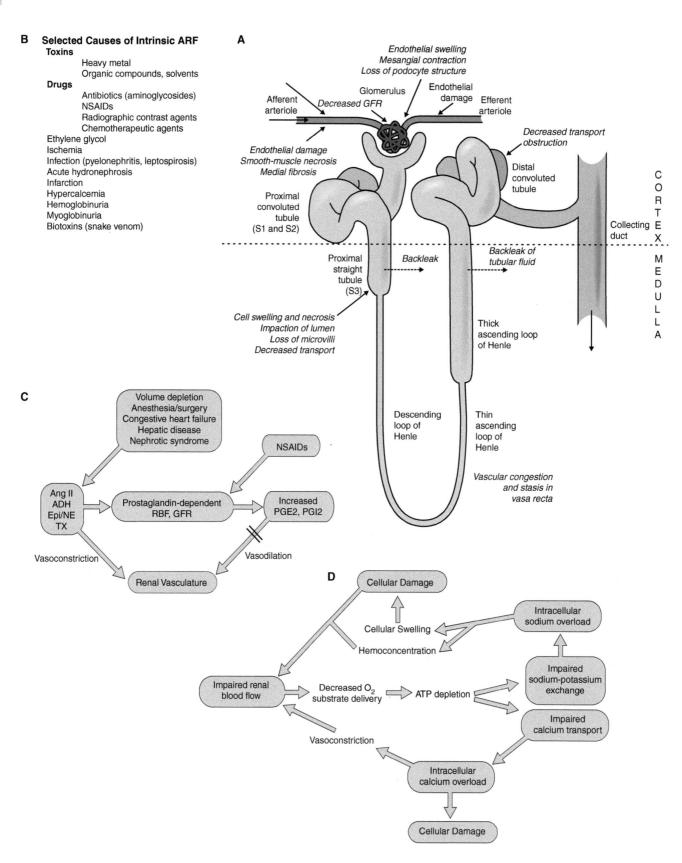

B Selected Causes of Intrinsic ARF
- Toxins
  - Heavy metal
  - Organic compounds, solvents
- Drugs
  - Antibiotics (aminoglycosides)
  - NSAIDs
  - Radiographic contrast agents
  - Chemotherapeutic agents
- Ethylene glycol
- Ischemia
- Infection (pyelonephritis, leptospirosis)
- Acute hydronephrosis
- Infarction
- Hypercalcemia
- Hemoglobinuria
- Myoglobinuria
- Biotoxins (snake venom)

Acute renal failure (ARF) is a syndrome characterized by abrupt deterioration of renal function with a resultant inability to regulate solute and water balance. ARF can be caused by acute prerenal failure, primary (intrinsic) failure, or postrenal failure. Intrinsic ARF occurs more frequently than is generally recognized and is often misdiagnosed as chronic renal failure. It is a tenuously reversible state, that must be diagnosed quickly and treated aggressively.

Pathophysiology

Acute tubular necrosis is a syndrome of abrupt and sustained reduction in GFR resulting from an ischemic or toxic renal insult and accounts for the majority of cases of primary (intrinsic) ARF. Three mechanisms may contribute to decreased GFR or reduced renal tubular flow rate during ARF: tubular obstruction, tubular backleak, and primary filtration failure (**Part A**). Tubular backleak occurs when filtrate leaks back across or between damaged tubular cells and enters the renal venous circulation. Primary filtration failure results from inadequate glomerular capillary plasma flow, inadequate glomerular hydrostatic pressure, or altered glomerular permeability.

Renal Hypoperfusion/Ischemia

The causes of hemodynamically mediated ARF are the same as those predisposing to prerenal ARF; the influences are more profound and prolonged in intensity and duration with intrinsic ARF (**Part B**). Hypotension, hypovolemia, circulatory collapse, or other causes of insufficient renal perfusion (e.g., renal artery infarcts, disseminated intravascular coagulation, vasculitis) can initiate ARF. Animals that have experienced hemorrhage, trauma, extensive surgery, or prolonged anesthesia are at increased risk for the development of ARF.

Intrarenal vasoconstriction is key to the development of ischemic ARF. In an attempt to maintain systemic arterial blood pressure during situations of hypoperfusion, increased vasopressor activity occurs as a result of increased activity of the sympathetic nervous system. The renal vasculature also experiences vasoconstriction from stimulation of renal catecholamine and angiotensin receptors. Under normal conditions or during brief episodes of hypoperfusion, this effect is counterbalanced by the intrarenal production of prostaglandins (**Part C**).

Renal vasoconstriction decreases renal blood flow in both the cortex and the medulla, with greater reductions in blood flow occurring in the cortex. Preservation of blood flow to the medulla may be a protective mechanism to supply oxygen to the metabolically active tubular cells in the outer medulla. Swelling of proximal tubular cells located in the outer medulla further reduces renal blood flow, potentiating ischemic injury to the thick ascending limb of Henle's loop (**Part D**). Renal tubular damage resulting from ischemia is characterized by a patchy distribution along nephrons, with a tendency toward disruption of the tubular basement membranes.

Infection

Sepsis or primary urinary tract infection is a common cause of ARF (**Part B**). Patients with acute pyelonephritis or leptospirosis have clinical signs that may vary from mild and nonspecific (pyrexia, lethargy, anorexia, vomiting) to profound (acute abdomen) consistent with septicemia.

Nephrotoxic Chemicals and Drugs

The administration of many chemicals and drugs has been associated with the development of ARF (see **Part B**). Renal injury is attributed to attachment of the toxic agent to luminal, basolateral, or intracellular organelle membranes of renal tubular and glomerular cells. Increased membrane permeability and loss of cellular functions occur. Excessive activation of the renin-angiotensin system results in a decrease in GFR and renal blood flow, which leads to tubular necrosis. The degradation of phospholipids in cell membranes appears to be central in initiating and perpetuating tubular cell injury. The role of intracellular calcium in the development of ischemic and nephrotoxic injury is unclear, but redistribution of calcium within the cell may be important in the early activation of phospholipase (see **Part D**).

NSAIDs are used widely in veterinary medicine for the treatment of arthritis and other inflammatory conditions. All NSAIDs inactivate cyclooxygenase, a major enzyme in the biosynthetic pathway of eicosanoids. ARF results primarily from inhibition of local eicosanoid (prostaglandin) synthesis (local regulators of renal blood flow and renal tubular function) (see **Part C**).

Ingestion of ethylene glycol (as antifreeze) is the most common cause of nephrotoxicity encountered in veterinary medical patients. The mortality rate is high. Successful treatment of the intoxicated patient hinges on a rapid diagnosis and early institution of therapy.

Ethylene glycol is rapidly absorbed from the GI tract and distributed to all body tissues. The metabolites (glycolaldehyde, glycolate, glyoxalate, oxalate) of ethylene glycol are responsible for its toxicity. Inhibition of alcohol dehydrogenase, the enzyme responsible for the first oxidative step in ethylene glycol metabolism, with administration of ethanol or 4-methylpyrazole results in the excretion of unmetabolized ethylene glycol by the kidneys and forms the basis for treatment. The minimum lethal dose of ethylene glycol is 4.2–6.6 mL/kg in dogs and 1.5 mL/kg in cats. Cats produce relatively large amounts of oxalate during the metabolism of ethylene glycol, which may account for their increased sensitivity.

Aminoglycoside nephrotoxicity is the second most common cause of ARF in dogs and cats. Aminoglycosides are eliminated almost exclusively by glomerular filtration. Active uptake of aminoglycosides by the proximal tubules leads to accumulation of these drugs within the cells. The aminoglycosides then interfere with mitochondrial function and with normal lysosomal maturation and turnover. Lysosomal phospholipase is inhibited. The result is accumulation of lysosomes within the cells and a decrease in cellular respiration resulting in acute tubular necrosis.

Phases

The incipient phase is the period from exposure to a nephrotoxin or ischemic event to when azotemia is detected or a change in volume of urine production is noted in the animal. The incipient phase usually goes undetected, as clinical signs are minimal. Prompt treatment of the inciting cause of injury, if detected during the incipient phase, will result in rapid return to normal renal function. The maintenance phase is the period when established ARF is readily apparent. During this phase azotemia will be progressive or constant despite the correction of prerenal factors. Treatment of the inciting cause will not result in an immediate return of normal renal function. This phase may last 7–14 days or may be longer. Serum creatinine and BUN levels reach plateau values; urine specific gravity remains isosthenuric, and oliguria may or may not be present. Examination of urine sediment may reveal an increased number of renal tubular casts and renal epithelial cells. The recovery phase is characterized by return of normal renal function and resolution of the renal lesions. The time from the beginning of recovery to complete recovery is variable. Residual defects in renal concentrating and acidifying functions may persist but usually are not of clinical consequence. Functional hypertrophy of single nephrons restores the GFR and renal blood flow to normal despite a smaller number of surviving nephrons.

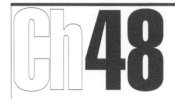

Acute Intrinsic Renal Failure II: Diagnosis

Robert J. Murtaugh

A

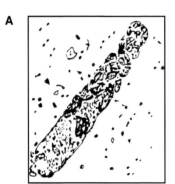

Cellular cast and fat droplets
(out of focus)

B

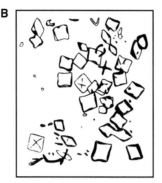

Calcium oxalate dihydrate

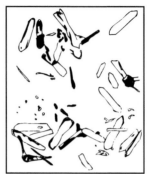

Calcium oxalate monohydrate

C   **Acute Renal Failure**

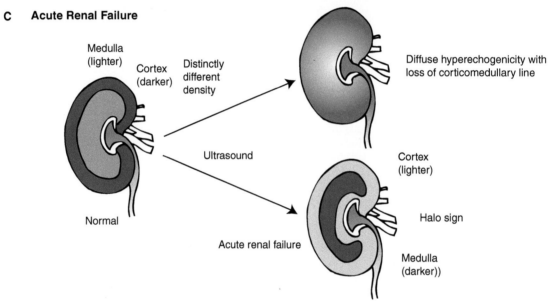

Medulla (lighter)

Cortex (darker)

Distinctly different density

Normal

Ultrasound

Acute renal failure

Diffuse hyperechogenicity with loss of corticomedullary line

Cortex (lighter)

Halo sign

Medulla (darker))

D   **Renal Biopsy**

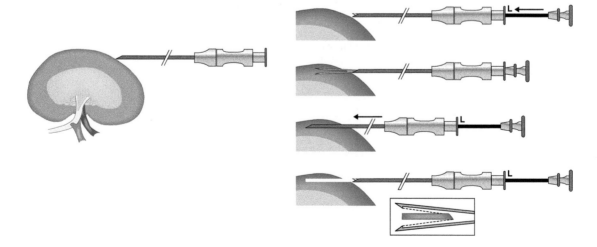

History

There is no age, breed, or sex predilection for intrinsic ARF. A history of recent trauma, surgical intervention, or anesthetic procedure may suggest the possibility of ischemic nephropathy. Recent administration of a known nephrotoxic drug may offer further evidence suggestive of intrinsic ARF. Access to ethylene glycol or actual observation of its ingestion is helpful in making that diagnosis.

Clinical Signs

Acute lethargy, anorexia, vomiting, diarrhea, and melena are common clinical signs. Animals with ARF do not produce a characteristic urine volume, although most of these animals are oliguric (<1 mL/kg/hr); anuria, polyuria, or normal urine volumes may be observed. Compared to oliguric ARF, nonoliguric ARF is thought to result from less severe renal injury.

A number of complications may be encountered with ARF. Loss of the ability to modify the character of the urine leads to disturbances in the volume and composition of body fluids. GI abnormalities are among the most common complications of ARF. Diffuse erosive gastritis, septic ulcer disease, or uremic colitis may develop. GI hemorrhage remains a major cause of morbidity and mortality in patients with ARF. Secondary infections occur in 40%–80% of human patients with intrinsic ARF, representing a second major cause of mortality. Data on the prevalence of these infections associated with ARF in veterinary patients are not available. Neurological complications of ARF (stupor, coma, seizure) usually are observed with ethylene glycol intoxication and as terminal events.

Physical Examination

Dogs and cats presenting with ARF are generally lethargic, hypovolemic, hyperpneic, bradycardiac, and hypothermic. The presence of fever may be supportive evidence for inflammatory or infectious renal disease. Abdominal palpation may reveal a small, normal, or large urinary bladder. Renal pain may be elicited. The kidneys, if palpable, should be of normal size or slightly enlarged. Chronic renal disease is suggested by small and irregular kidneys.

Laboratory Testing

A complete blood cell count may reveal a leukocytosis (secondary to stress or infection). The red blood cell count is variable—either elevated secondary to dehydration or decreased secondary to hemorrhage, hemolysis, or hemodilution. Bleeding time and values for other parameters of platelet function are abnormal. A number of different factors may contribute to the bleeding diathesis seen with ARF; these include a direct effect on platelet function by urea or guanidinosuccinic acid, reduced platelet factor 3 activity, abnormal capillary integrity, and increased prostacyclin (PGI_2) synthesis.

The serum biochemical profile will reveal elevated BUN, serum phosphorus, and serum creatinine levels. Hyperkalemia will be evident in animals with oliguric ARF. Serum calcium concentration may be normal, low, or elevated depending on the cause of the ARF. Ethylene glycol–induced ARF may result in severe (symptomatic) hypocalcemia, as calcium is chelated from the plasma by oxalate metabolites of ethylene glycol. Serum sodium concentrations can be normal, low, or elevated depending on the factors contributing to patient dehydration and the stage of the disease process.

Abnormalities in acid-base balance should be evaluated by blood gas analysis. A moderate to severe metabolic acidosis is usually present. The finding of simultaneous large serum anion and osmolal gaps early in the course is helpful in supporting a diagnosis of ARF due to ethylene glycol intoxication. Measurement of ethylene glycol concentration in whole blood, serum, or urine within 12 hours of poisoning using an ethylene glycol test kit (PRN Pharmacal) is helpful in confirming the diagnosis.

If urine is being produced, urinalysis should be performed and urine should be submitted for bacteriological culture and antibiotic sensitivity testing. Urine specific gravity is in the isosthenuria range (1,007–1,015), and proteinuria, hematuria, and glucosuria are evident. Glucosuria despite normoglycemia, and alkaline urine despite systemic metabolic acidosis are indicative of proximal tubular damage typical of acute tubular necrosis. The urine sediment should be evaluated for evidence of bacteria, red blood cells, white blood cells, casts, and crystals (**Part A**). Acute tubular necrosis and nephritis may result in the formation of significant numbers of renal tubular casts. The presence of calcium oxalate dihydrate or monohydrate (hippurate) crystals in the urinary sediment of an animal with ARF supports a diagnosis of ethylene glycol poisoning (**Part B**).

Diagnostic Imaging

Radiographic and ultrasonographic evaluation of the kidney is not generally helpful in the diagnosis of ARF. The main indication is to aid in ruling out chronic renal disease. In ARF, radiographic or ultrasonographic examination of the kidneys should demonstrate normal or enlarged renal size and shape (**Part C**). Altered corticomedullary echogenicity and loss of distinction between the renal cortex and medulla also can be evident ultrasonographically. In dogs and cats with marked azotemia and oliguria, the excretory urogram rarely provides diagnostic information.

Renal Biopsy

Histopathological examination of renal biopsy specimens can demonstrate lesions compatible with ARF, including degenerative tubular changes, tubular necrosis, desquamation of tubular cells, denuding and disruption of tubular basement membranes, and intrarenal cast formation. Renal biopsy is helpful in evaluating for the presence of intact basement membranes, adequate tubular regeneration and repopulation of tubular cells, or significant fibrosis and nephron loss (**Part D**). The prognosis is particularly important when expense and effort must be justified in relation to the potential reversibility of the injury. Bacteriological cultures of renal tissue should be grown to rule in or rule out an infectious cause of ARF. Silver stains may be useful in diagnosing the presence of spirochete organisms (leptospirosis). The diagnosis of glomerulonephritides may require electron microscopy.

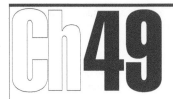

Acute Intrinsic Renal Failure III: Treatment

Robert J. Murtaugh

A Treatment of Ethylene Glycol Intoxication

Ethanol administration

Dogs:

5.5 mL of 20% ethanol/kg IV every 4 or 5 treatments, then every 6 hours for 4 treatments

0.6 gm of 7% ethanol/kg IV as a bolus, followed by 100 mg/kg/hr as a continous IV infusion continued until 10 hr postdialysis (see below)

Cats:

5 mL of 20% ethanol/kg IV every 6 hr for 5 treatments, then every 8 hr for 4 treatments

4-Methylpyrazole-dogs only
20 mg of a 5% solution/kg IV initially, followed by a 15 mg/kg IV at 12 hr and 24 hr, and 5 mg/kg IV at 36 hr after the first dose

Peritoneal dialysis
For acute removal of ethylene glycol [multiple exchanges using 1.5% dextrose concentration dialysate (20 mL/kg/exchange)] continuing until 8 hr after correction of metabolic acidosis

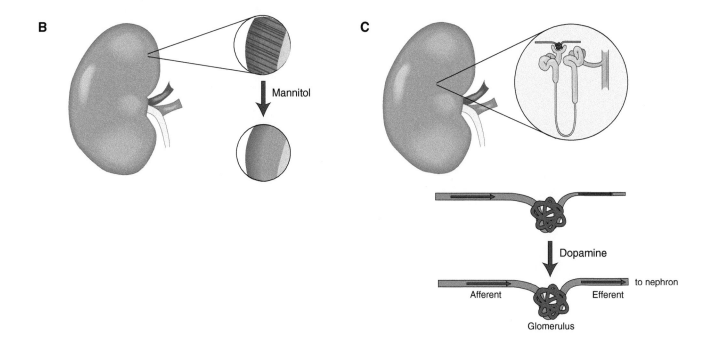

Therapy for intrinsic ARF can be divided into conservative medical management and dialysis. The basic aims for established ARF are to correct the renal hemodynamic disorders and alleviate the fluid and biochemical abnormalities until renal repair can take place. The administration of antidotal treatment is indicated for incipient ARF following ethylene glycol intoxication (**Part A**).

Fluid Therapy

There are 2 main objectives of fluid therapy: 1) correction of fluid, acid-base, and electrolyte imbalances; and 2) initiation or augmentation of diuresis to improve renal function and enhance excretion of metabolic waste products and uremic toxins.

It is extremely important to assess and continually reassess body weight, packed cell volume, total serum solid levels, skin turgor, central venous pressure, and urine production (indwelling urinary catheter), as changes in these parameters form the basis for calculation of fluid, acid-base, and electrolyte requirements.

Initial fluid therapy should consist of IV administration of a balanced electrolyte solution. The type of fluid administered should be dictated by serum sodium levels. Dehydration in animals with suspected ARF should be corrected more rapidly than in animals with normal renal function, to prevent further renal damage from ischemia and to differentiate physiological oliguria from pathological oliguria. Measurement of central venous pressure may be necessary for monitoring fluid administration, to prevent overhydration in oliguric patients. In the case of physiological oliguria, urine flow should increase to 2–5 mL/kg/hr depending on the rate of fluid administration. If adequate urine production has not been established following rehydration, therapy with diuretics and vasoactive drugs to restore urine production is indicated.

Diuretics

Diuretic administration is indicated in the management of pathological oliguria. Furosemide (2.2 mg/kg IV) is the diuretic of choice. Urine production should increase within 30 minutes following administration of furosemide, or the dose can be doubled or tripled at hourly intervals. However, bolus doses >5 mg/kg seem to have no additional benefit. A continuous IV infusion of furosemide (0.5 mg/kg/hr) can be utilized following initial IV bolus administration.

An osmotic diuretic can be tried if furosemide administration fails to increase urine production (mannitol 0.5–1.0gm/kg infused over 15–20 minutes) (**Part B**). Urine production should begin within 15–30 minutes if the treatment is effective. Mannitol administration is contraindicated in the overhydrated oliguric animal.

Vasoactive Drugs

Dopamine is the vasodilator most often used in conjunction with furosemide to augment renal function and urine production in oliguric animals. Dopamine administration reduces renal vascular resistance and increases renal blood flow, particularly in the inner renal cortex (**Part C**). The effects are mediated through dopaminergic receptors in the renal vasculature. Dopamine is diluted in an isotonic fluid and administered IV at a rate of 2–5 µg/kg/min. Dopamine is arrhythmogenic, and animals receiving an IV infusion of it should be monitored electrocardiographically.

If oliguria persists despite the use of aggressive treatment with IV fluid, diuretic, and vasodilator administration, peritoneal dialysis or hemodialysis will be necessary.

Management of Acid-Base and Electrolyte Abnormalities

Refer to Chapter 1–17 for specific therapeutic approaches to these conditions.

A moderate to severe metabolic acidosis is the most common acid-base problem seen with ARF, and the most significant electrolyte abnormality associated with ARF is hyperkalemia. Hypercalcemia is encountered infrequently with ARF but has been associated with neoplasia and rodenticide intoxication. Hypocalcemia may be observed with ARF but is usually mild to moderate and asymptomatic. Severe hypocalcemia resulting in tetany may be seen with ethylene glycol intoxication and severe crushing injuries. Hyperphosphatemia occurs commonly with ARF because of the decrease in GFR.

For prolonged control of hyperkalemia in patients with oliguric renal failure, a cationic exchange resin, sodium polystyrene sulfonate, can be administered orally at 2 gm/kg/day in 3 divided doses. Effective long-term control of hyperkalemia is obtained with dialysis.

Hypokalemia (potassium level <3.5 mEq/l) may occur with overcorrection of hyperkalemic states and in conjunction with decreased intake. It also may occur with nonoliguric ARF due to renal potassium losses. Hypokalemia is most prevalent with gentamicin-induced ARF and with the recovery phase of acute tubular necrosis.

Abnormalities in serum sodium levels (hyponatremia or hypernatremia) may occur with ARF. Serum sodium levels should be assessed at least once daily, and appropriate changes made in the type of fluid therapy administered.

Acute Intrinsic Renal Failure IV: Peritoneal Dialysis Treatment

Robert J. Murtaugh

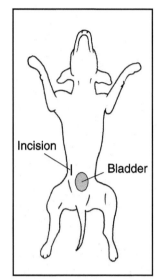

Incision

Bladder

Catheter device comes out of belly to right of ventral midline and is angled into caudal fossa alongside bladder.

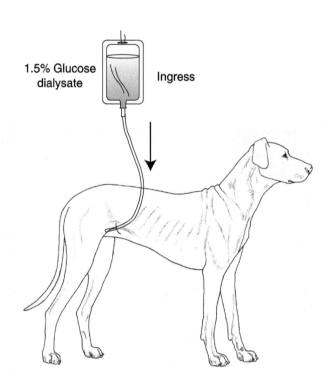

1.5% Glucose dialysate

Ingress

Time frame = 1 hour

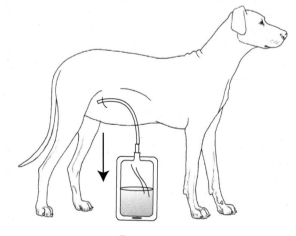

Egress

Dialysis

When intensive fluid therapy and diuretic administration do not reestablish urine flow or improve renal function, dialysis is indicated. Dialysis is the recommended treatment for patients with reversible ARF (aminoglycoside- or ethylene glycol–induced ARF). Dialysis is a labor-intensive treatment and therefore is expensive. When ARF is due to a reversible toxic insult, when it is detected early, or when renal biopsy establishes a good prognosis, then dialysis is a treatment worth considering. Dialysis can be used to correct acid-base and electrolyte imbalances, remove the toxic agent and other metabolic waste products, and maintain the animal until renal tissue has regenerated. Peritoneal dialysis is the most common approach for dialysis in veterinary medicine and involves use of the peritoneum as a semipermeable membrane for the exchange of water and solute.

Peritoneal Dialysis

Aseptic technique is imperative with any type of peritoneal dialysis. This includes the use of surgical scrub and sterile surgical techniques during catheter placement, as well as the use of sterile gloves, disinfectants, and the careful handling of dialysate fluids, catheters, and catheter lines during dialysis (**Figure**).

Access to the Peritoneal Cavity

Several types of catheters are available for performing peritoneal dialysis. Selection of a particular catheter will depend on the duration of dialysis anticipated and the number of daily exchanges of dialysate prescribed to manage an animal's uremia. Animals with severe adhesions along the midline or those with ileus will require a surgically placed catheter.

Selection and Preparation of Dialysate

Dialysate generally is chosen to approximate normal plasma composition (with the exception of proteins). Dialysate should be tailored, however, to the individual patient for sodium, chloride, potassium, and alkali needs. The concentration gradient between blood and dialysate largely determines what substances are removed from or added to the animal's blood. A large concentration gradient from blood to dialysate favors solute removal from the body, whereas a large concentration gradient from dialysate to blood favors uptake of solute to the body. The concentration gradient between blood and dialysate should be nonexistent for substances not desired to be removed from or added to the body.

Commercial Dialysate Solution

Commercially available peritoneal dialysis solutions designed for use in humans work well in dogs and cats. These polyelectrolyte peritoneal dialysis solutions approximate normal plasma electrolyte concentrations and contain dextrose at 1.5%, 2.5%, and 4.5% concentrations. Dialysate containing 1.5% dextrose is usually effective, but 2.5% or 4.5% dextrose solutions may be needed to correct overhydration or when effluent dialysate volume declines because of marked hyperosmolality of patient serum. Hypernatremia occurs commonly during peritoneal dialysis and is attributed to ultrafiltration of solute-free water. For this reason it may be advantageous or necessary to choose dialysate solutions that are lower in sodium concentration than plasma during the course of dialysis.

Prewarming Dialysate

Prewarming of dialysate is recommended when exchanges are conducted frequently during aggressive dialysis (every 1–3 hours). Fluids 1–2°C higher than body temperature have been recommended in an effort to vasodilate the peritoneal vasculature to enhance solute exchange.

Infusion of Dialysate

Rapid infusion of dialysate at 200–300 mL/min by gravity flow is well tolerated by animals. Infusion volumes of 250, 500, 1,000, and 2,000 mL are often chosen based on body weight to approximate a dose of 40 mL/kg. The abdomen should be palpably distended following dialysate infusion to ensure maximal contact of fluid with peritoneal surfaces.

Dwell Time for Dialysate

Dwell time for the dialysate is based on the urgency of need to correct uremic abnormalities. Animals with life-threatening conditions such as hyperkalemia and metabolic acidosis may require hourly exchanges until stabilization has occurred. Animals with ARF may require 12–48 consecutive hourly exchanges before a marked decline in uremic solute (BUN, serum creatinine, serum phosphorus) can be demonstrated.

Drainage of Effluent

Dialysate is drained by gravity usually within 15 minutes following an appropriate dwell time. It is best to drain effluent into the same bag used to infuse dialysate so that chances for bacterial contamination are minimized during manipulations of the mechanical apparatus. Effluent volume should closely match or exceed the volume infused during subsequent hourly exchanges with 1.5% dextrose solutions.

Failure to retrieve 90% or more of the infused dialysate following hourly exchanges usually indicates a mechanical problem with drainage.

Occasionally, reduced effluent volume is the result of increased peritoneal absorption of fluid and solute. This can follow marked dehydration (low capillary hydrostatic pressure), increased plasma osmolality, or increased plasma protein concentration (increased oncotic pressure) such that fluid absorption into the blood vessels is favored.

Ancillary Treatments

Vomiting, hematemesis, melena, and anorexia must be addressed. Histamine (H_2) receptor blockers have been recommended for control of uremic gastritis and ulcers. Vomiting associated with ARF may be severe and persistent. The thorazine tranquilizers act as centrally acting antiemetics and seem to ameliorate nausea and vomiting in animals with ARF.

Animals in ARF are in a hypercatabolic state and nutritional support is indicated. The supply of calories helps decrease the catabolic response, lessening the degree of protein breakdown products requiring renal excretion. Additionally, regeneration of renal tubular cells requires an extensive supply of energy and protein. By considering these demands early in the course of treatment of animals with ARF, complications (weight loss, increased risk of infection, decubital ulcers) may be avoided.

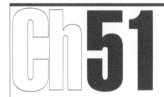

Congestive Heart Failure I: Diastolic Dysfunction

Maureen McMichael

A

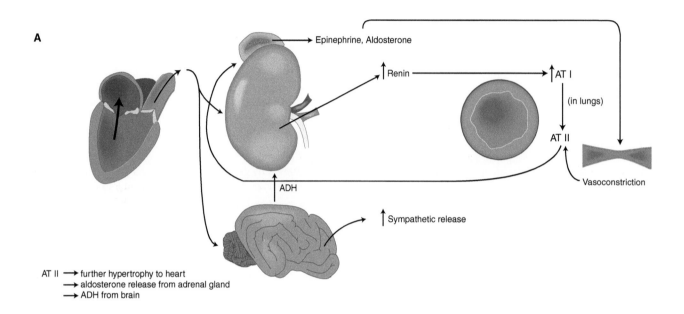

Epinephrine, Aldosterone

↑ Renin

↑ AT I

(in lungs)

AT II

Vasoconstriction

ADH

↑ Sympathetic release

AT II ⟶ further hypertrophy to heart
⟶ aldosterone release from adrenal gland
⟶ ADH from brain

B

Normal Heart   Diastolic Dysfunction

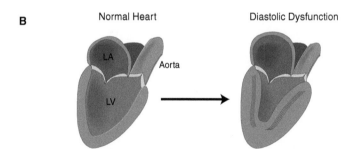

LA

Aorta

LV

When cardiac output decreases, whether due to decreased ventricular filling (diastolic dysfunction), diminished contractility (systolic dysfunction), mechanical restriction (restrictive cardiomyopathy), or valvular disease, several neurohumoral compensatory mechanisms are triggered to attempt to restore cardiac function.

Of these mechanisms, activation of the sympathetic nervous system and the renin-angiotensin-aldosterone system has the most significant effect. The sympathetic nervous system causes an increase in heart rate, cardiac contractility, and peripheral vasoconstriction. Renal juxtaglomerular cells release renin in response to decreased renal perfusion. Renin converts angiotensinogen to angiotensin I. Angiotensin I is converted to angiotensin II by angiotensin-converting enzyme (ACE).

Angiotensin II is 1 of the most potent vasoconstrictors known (**Part A**) and preferentially constricts renal efferent arterioles to a greater degree than renal afferent arterioles in an attempt to increase renal perfusion. Angiotensin II also causes release of aldosterone, which increases sodium reabsorption in the collecting ducts, and antidiuretic hormone (ADH), which increases reabsorption of water from the renal collecting ducts. Angiotensin II also directly causes sodium retention by renal tubules and increased norepinephrine release along with vascular wall and myocardial cell hypertrophy.

In the early stages of congestive heart failure (CHF), these compensatory mechanisms restore cardiac output and maintain circulatory volume. In more advanced stages of cardiac disease, the vasoconstriction (increased afterload) and increase in preload (increased volume from sodium and water retention) overwhelm the failing heart and lead to CHF. In left-sided heart failure, pulmonary edema predominates, and in right-sided heart failure, pleural effusion, ascites, jugular venous distention, and hepatomegaly are typically present.

Diastolic Dysfunction

Pathophysiology

Animals with diastolic dysfunction (**Part B**) have a primary impairment in ventricular relaxation. This impaired relaxation interferes with normal cardiac filling. Feline hypertrophic cardiomyopathy (HCM) is an example of diastolic dysfunction. Several gross and histological findings seen in cats with HCM include concentric left ventricular (LV) hypertrophy, increased ventricular wall stiffness, interventricular septal hypertrophy, myocardial fibrosis and ischemia, narrowed LV outflow tract, fibrosis and thickening of the mitral valve, and left atrial (LA) dilatation. Histologically, hypertrophied and degenerative myocytes with enlarged nuclei and varying degrees of endocardial and interstitial fibrosis are observed. A genetic basis in Maine coon cats and Persians has been proposed.

Impaired LV filling and cardiac output result from a combination of increased LV stiffness (causing decreased compliance), myocardial hypertrophy (increased wall thickness), and fibrosis. Decreased cardiac output stimulates the baroreceptors (through decreased blood pressure), the sympathetic nervous system is activated, and ADH is released. Decreased renal perfusion activates the renin-angiotensin-aldosterone system. Impaired LV filling leads to elevations in LV end-diastolic pressure. LA pressure must rise in order to fill the LV during diastole, and the elevated LA pressure is transmitted backward, resulting in elevated pulmonary venous pressures and pulmonary edema. Chronic left-sided heart failure may lead to pulmonary arterial hypertension and right-sided heart failure.

Clinical Signs and Presentation

Most cats with HCM and CHF present with weakness, tachypnea, dyspnea, and tachycardia. Delayed capillary refill time, pale or cyanotic mucous membranes, weak arterial pulses, and harsh lung sounds or pulmonary crackles often are observed in these cats. A gallop rhythm or a cardiac murmur may be present on auscultation. Jugular pulses will often be observed, especially in cats with biventricular CHF and pleural effusion.

Diagnosis

Definitive diagnosis of HCM is made by echocardiography, thoracic radiography, and ECG. Echocardiographic findings include hypertrophy of the LV and dilatation of the LA. Radiographic findings may include pulmonary venous distention, interstitial to alveolar pulmonary edema, pleural effusion, and an enlarged cardiac silhouette with an enlarged LA or biatrial enlargement (the valentine heart on VD views). ECG findings may indicate sinus tachycardia, atrial or ventricular arrhythmias, and left-sided heart enlargement by left-axis deviation to the QRS complex, increased P-wave duration, or increased QRS duration or amplitude. Hyperthyroidism and systemic hypertension are differential diagnoses that can mimic idiopathic HCM in cats. A complete blood cell count, serum biochemical profile, urinalysis, systemic arterial blood pressure measurement, and a serum T_4 analysis (in any cat >6 years old) should be performed to obtain a minimum data base in cats with suspected HCM.

Treatment

It is essential that these cats be treated with a minimum of stress. Cats that present severely dyspneic are placed in a quiet oxygenated (40% FIO_2) environment after an injection of furosemide (4 mg/kg IV) and an application of nitroglycerin paste ($1/8$–$1/4$ inch placed on a shaved or hairless area). These treatments are repeated in 1–2 hours if necessary and continued at tapering intervals in association with the resolution of the clinical signs of CHF. If lung sounds are dull ventrally on auscultation and jugular distention is present, a therapeutic thoracocentesis is performed for removal of suspected pleural effusion.

When the dyspnea has resolved and the cat appears more comfortable, further definitive diagnostic tests can be performed. Chronic treatment includes the administration of enalapril (1.25–2.50 mg PO q24h), sustained-release diltiazem (30 mg PO q24h), and furosemide (1 mg/kg PO qod–bid) as needed to control signs of congestion.

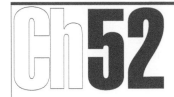

Congestive Heart Failure II: Systolic Dysfunction

Maureen McMichael

A

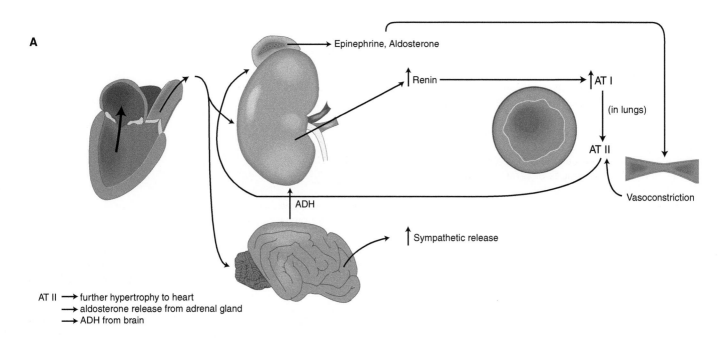

Epinephrine, Aldosterone

↑Renin

↑AT I

(in lungs)

AT II

Vasoconstriction

ADH

↑Sympathetic release

AT II ⟶ further hypertrophy to heart
⟶ aldosterone release from adrenal gland
⟶ ADH from brain

B

Normal Heart   Systolic Dysfunction

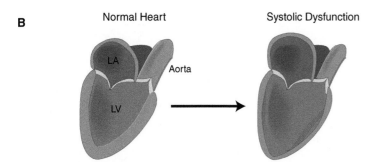

LA

Aorta

LV

When cardiac output decreases, whether due to decreased ventricular filling (diastolic dysfunction), diminished contractility (systolic dysfunction), mechanical restriction (restrictive cardiomyopathy), or valvular disease, several neurohumoral compensatory mechanisms are triggered to attempt to restore cardiac function.

Of these mechanisms, activation of the sympathetic nervous system and the renin-angiotensin-aldosterone system has the most significant effect. The sympathetic nervous system causes an increase in heart rate, cardiac contractility, and peripheral vasoconstriction. Renal juxtaglomerular cells release renin in response to decreased renal perfusion. Renin converts angiotensinogen to angiotensin I. Angiotensin I is converted to angiotensin II by angiotensin-converting enzyme (ACE).

Angiotensin II is 1 of the most potent vasoconstrictors known (**Part A**) and preferentially constricts renal efferent arterioles to a greater degree than renal afferent arterioles in an attempt to increase renal perfusion. Angiotensin II also causes release of aldosterone, which increases sodium reabsorption in the collecting ducts, and antidiuretic hormone (ADH), which increases reabsorption of water from the renal collecting ducts. Angiotensin II also directly causes sodium retention by renal tubules and increased norepinephrine release along with vascular wall and myocardial cell hypertrophy.

In the early stages of congestive heart failure (CHF), these compensatory mechanisms restore cardiac output and maintain circulatory volume. In more advanced stages of cardiac disease, the vasoconstriction (increased afterload) and increase in preload (increased volume from sodium and water retention) overwhelm the failing heart and lead to CHF. In left-sided heart failure, pulmonary edema predominates, and in right-sided heart failure, pleural effusion, ascites, jugular venous distention, and hepatomegaly are typically present.

Systolic Dysfunction

Pathophysiology

In animals with systolic cardiac dysfunction (**Part B**), there is a primary inability of the myocardium to contract effectively, leading to initiation of the compensatory pathophysiological spiral of CHF development described previously. Canine dilated cardiomyopathy (DCM) is an example of this type of dysfunction. There is a breed predilection for Doberman pinschers, boxers, and American cocker spaniels. Large-breed dogs are affected more commonly than are small breeds. Gross and histological changes may include marked dilatation of the LA and LV (or in some cases, of all of the chambers), thickening of the endocardium, valvular degeneration, atrophy of the papillary muscles, myocardial fibrosis and degeneration, and myocyte atrophy. The disease is idiopathic in most patients, but reduced levels of L-carnitine have been found in myocytes in a small percentage of boxers and reduced plasma and myocardial levels of taurine in some cocker spaniels with DCM. Supplementation of these nutraceuticals has resulted in reversal of disease in some of these instances.

Clinical Signs and Presentation

At presentation, dogs with DCM and low-output failure often are weak or collapsed with weak arterial pulses, pale to cyanotic mucous membranes, jugular distention, cold extremities, and palpable ascites. A cardiac murmur (usually due to mitral or tricuspid insufficiency) may be auscultated along with an S_3 gallop and cardiac arrhythmias. In animals with CHF and DCM, lung auscultation may reveal crackles (pulmonary edema) or quiet lung sounds (pleural effusion). Jugular vein distention is often present.

Diagnosis

Definitive diagnosis of DCM is made with echocardiographic examination. Fractional shortening (percentage change in LV lumen dimension between diastole and systole), as a measure of the effective contractility of the myocardium, is decreased. Normal fractional shortening is >30%, and dogs with DCM often have values as low as 10%–20%.

Thoracic radiographs may show an enlarged cardiac silhouette, an enlarged LA, and enlarged pulmonary veins with interstitial to alveolar pulmonary edema. With right-sided CHF, an enlarged caudal vena cava, pleural effusion, hepatomegaly, and ascites may be observed on radiographs.

ECG findings may include sinus tachycardia (heart rate >160 bpm), wide P waves (>0.04–0.05 second, suggesting LA enlargement), wide QRS complexes (>0.06 second), and tall R waves (>3 mV in lead II, suggesting LV enlargement). Atrial fibrillation (no P waves, an irregularly irregular QRS rhythm) with ventricular premature complexes and various conduction disturbances such as atrioventricular and bundle branch blocks are often observed on ECG.

Prerenal azotemia from decreased renal perfusion and a mild elevation in liver enzyme levels from hepatic congestion often are observed on serum biochemistry studies of patients with DCM.

Treatment

Improving contractility and increasing cardiac output, decreasing pulmonary edema, and managing cardiac arrhythmias are the main goals of treatment. Emergency resuscitation of animals with DCM includes administration of oxygen (nasal oxygen or oxygen cage), furosemide (4 mg/kg IV, IM, q1–3h) to eliminate pulmonary edema, and dobutamine infusion (2–10 μg/kg/min). Dobutamine is a synthetic catecholamine used to increase cardiac inotropy without significantly increasing heart rate. Specific antiarrhythmic therapies are described in Chapter 53 and 54.

Dobutamine is administered as a continuous-rate infusion as it has a half-life of 2–3 minutes. Successful clinical end points with dobutamine treatment are an increased systolic arterial blood pressure with improved mucous membrane color and capillary refill time. If the heart rate increases by 20% compared to the pretreatment rate, or worsening cardiac arrhythmias develop, the dobutamine infusion should be slowed or discontinued. Dobutamine administration is preferred over dopamine because dobutamine has less propensity to elevate the heart rate.

Chronic maintenance treatment for animals with DCM includes administration of ACE inhibitor therapy (0.5 mg/kg q12–24h), furosemide (1–4 mg/kg PO q8–12h), digoxin (0.005 mg/kg PO bid), and in selected cases L-carnitine and taurine supplementation. Treatment with additional antiarrhythmic drugs may be required based on ECG findings. The prognosis for survival with treatment for patients with DCM that respond to resuscitative therapy is generally measured in terms of weeks to months.

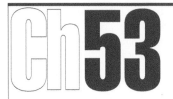

Cardiac Arrhythmias I: Recognition and Treatment

Maureen McMichael

A   **Sinus Tachycardia**

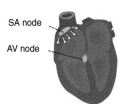

SA node

AV node

Definition/Recognition
Adult dog HR>180 bpm
Adult cat HR>240 bpm
Normal PQRST complexes

Causes
Anemia
Hypovolemia
Shock/Hypertension
Hyperthermia
Pain/fear
Catecholamines
(pheochromocytoma)
Hyperthyroidism
Toxins (e.g. theobromine)

Treatment
Usually not necessary
Treat underlying cause
Vagal maneuvers (carotid sinus
or ocular pressure) may
gradually and temporarily
decrease rate; can help
differentiate sinus
tachycardia from
supraventricular tachycardia

B   **Sinus Bradycardia**

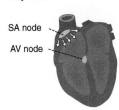

SA node

AV node

Definition/Recognition
HR < 70 bpm (dog)
HR < 140 bpm (cat)
Normal PQRST morphology

Causes
Intracranial Pressure (ICP)
Hypothermia
Hyperkalemia
Drugs and toxins
High vagal tone
(GI or respiratory diseases)

Treatment
Not usually needed
Treat the underlying cause
If head trauma present, check BP,
if hypertensive, consider mannitol
to decrease ICP

C   **Hyperkalemia**

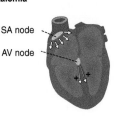

SA node

AV node

Definition/Recognition
Peaked T wave and slow HR
seen 1st then
P-wave amplitude decreases
and see wide QRS-
sinoventricular conduction

Causes
Urethral obstruction
Acute renal failure (ARF)
Hypoadrenocorticism

Treatment
1. Stat K^+ level
2. NaCl 0.9% bolus 1/4-1/2 shock dose
3. Calcium gluconate 0.5 mL/kg slow IV
4. Unblock if obstructed
5. Consider furosemide and dopamine for ARF
6. Consider colloids for hypoadrenocorticism
and dexamethasone

D   **Sick Sinus Syndrome**

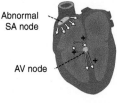

Abnormal
SA node

AV node

Definition/Recognition
Usually small-breed canine
(especiallly mini-schnauzer)
Can see sinus bradycardia,
sinus arrest and/or SVT
Often runs of bradycardia
followed by runs of tachycardia

Causes
Abnormalities of sinus node

Treatment
1. Pacemaker implantation is
treatment of choice
2. If only bradycardia seen, can
try atropine 0.04 mg/kg IV as diagnostic step
3. If tachycardia and bradycardia,
need pacemaker first, then can
try medication for tachycardia

E   **AV Block**

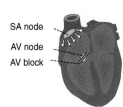

SA node

AV node

AV block

Definition/Recognition
HR < 70 bpm (dog)
HR < 140 bpm (cat)
Normal PQRST morphology

Causes
↑Intracranial Pressure (ICP)
Hypothermia
Hyperkalemia
Drugs and toxins
High vagal tone (GI diseases)

Treatment
Not usually needed
Treat the underlying cause
If head trauma present, check BP,
if hypertensive, consider mannitol
to decrease ICP

The normal depolarization of the heart occurs from the sinoatrial node and is conducted through the atrioventricular (AV) node to depolarize the ventricles. This process is assessed through examination of the PQRST complexes recorded on a surface ECG (**Part A**). Cardiac arrhythmias arise from an abnormal rhythmicity or shift of a pacemaker, blocks or abnormal pathways of impulse transmission, or spontaneous generation of abnormal impulses in any area of the heart. The primary questions to ask regarding whether treatment of an arrhythmia in a specific patient is warranted are as follows: 1) Is the arrhythmia causing clinical signs? 2) Is there primary cardiac disease in this patient or is extracardiac disease causing the arrhythmia? 3) Is the arrhythmia likely to cause further deterioration or death in the patient?

Abnormalities of Sinus Rhythm

Sinus Tachycardia
(More than 180 bpm in an adult dog and less than 240 bpm in an adult cat; see **Part A**).

There are several causes of sinus tachycardia, including hyperthermia, increased sympathetic tone (e.g., heart failure, pain, anxiety, etc.), hypovolemia, and toxins (e.g., theobromine). Treatment is directed at removing or alleviating the underlying cause of the increased heart rate.

Sinus Bradycardia
(More than 60 bpm in an adult dog and more than 120 bpm in an adult cat; **Part B**).

The resting heart rate varies greatly for different animals depending on body weight and fitness. An athletic greyhound can have a resting heart rate of 40 bpm and may be perfectly healthy, whereas a stressed cat with a heart rate of 140 bpm would have significant bradycardia. As with sinus tachycardia, treatment of sinus bradycardia is usually directed at the underlying cause such as a metabolic disorder, CNS disease, hypothermia, and toxin ingestion.

Sinus Arrhythmia
The variation in signals from the medullary respiratory center into the vasomotor center of the brain during inspiration and expiration causes alternating increases and decreases in the number of impulses transmitted to the heart through the sympathetic and vagus nerves. The result is a slowing of the heart rate on inspiration and an increase in heart rate during expiration. Sinus arrhythmia can be normal in dogs and occasionally in cats. The presence of an exaggerated sinus arrhythmia can indicate airway disease in an animal with coughing or dyspnea. As sinus arrhythmia is a normal cardiac rhythm or is observed in association with noncardiac disease, specific antiarrhythmic treatment usually is not required.

Supraventricular Conduction Disturbances

Atrial Standstill
The hallmark ECG features of atrial standstill are an absence of P-wave activity and QRS complexes that may appear normal (AV node origin) or wide and bizarre (ventricular origin) (**Part C**). The heart rate will vary considerably depending on the origin of the escape rhythm

(40–120 bpm in dogs, 90–160 bpm in cats). The most common causes include hyperkalemia, drug intoxication, or primary atrial myopathies. The treatment for hyperkalemia involves identification and elimination of the inciting cause along with emergent IV administration of glucose and regular, crystalline insulin or sodium bicarbonate to drive potassium into the intracellular fluid space. Pacemaker implantation is indicated for the treatment of primary (atrial myopathy) atrial standstill.

Sinus Arrest and Sick Sinus Syndrome (SSS)
This idiopathic functional and structural degeneration of nodal tissue (**Part D**) was first recognized in the miniature Schnauzer breed and has subsequently been identified in several other small-breed dogs (generally females). The common clinical manifestation observed is syncope, usually attributable to periods of sinus arrest. A variety of ECG abnormalities including sinus bradycardia, sinus arrest, paroxysmal supraventricular tachycardia, and concomitant AV nodal dysfunction can be observed. During the recording of an ECG in an animal with SSS it is common to detect paroxysms of bradycardia followed by runs of tachycardia. This disease can be difficult to treat medically as the treatment indicated for supraventricular tachycardia can exacerbate bradycardia and vice versa. Pacemaker implantation is the treatment of choice, although many animals will respond, at least partially or temporarily, to treatment with anticholinergic medication (see AV Block).

AV Block (Part E)
The causes of AV block include ischemia, inflammation (e.g., bacterial endocarditis), fibrosis or calcification of the AV node, marked parasympathetic stimulation, and toxicities.

- First-degree AV block. The ECG manifestation of first-degree AV block is a prolonged PR interval (>140 msec in dogs, >80 msec in cats). This represents a delay of conduction from the atrium to the ventricle, often from excess vagal tone, and no treatment is necessary.
- Second-degree AV block, types I and II. Type I second-degree AV block manifests electrocardiographically as a progressively longer PR interval until a P wave occurs without a QRS complex. Type II is associated with a constant PR interval with intermittent P waves without an accompanying QRS complex. Type II second-degree AV block is usually indicative of more severe underlying disease and may progress to third-degree (complete) AV block. Clinical manifestations of second-degree AV block can range from no clinical signs to frequent syncopal events. Treatment usually is directed at the underlying cause along with anticholinergic administration (propantheline 1–2 mg/kg PO tid) or pacemaker implantation.
- Third-degree (complete) AV block. With complete AV block, P waves are not associated with the QRS complexes. The heart is pacing with a ventricular escape rhythm (40 bpm in dogs, 100 bpm in cats). Animals with complete AV block can present with clinical signs of right-sided heart failure or syncope and collapse related to the bradyarrhythmia. Emergency pacemaker implantation is the recommended treatment.

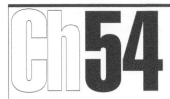

Cardiac Arrhythmias II: Recognition and Treatment

Maureen McMichael

A Atrial Premature Contractions

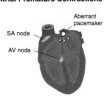

Definition/Recognition
P wave differs from sinus P wave; may be negative suggesting junctional origin
QRS is usually unaffected and resembles sinus QRS

Causes
Atrial dilation
Atrial irritation from ischemia, infection, toxins, thrombi, neoplasia, K+, digitalis

Treatment
Not usually necessary
Treat the underlying cardiac disease or other cause

B Supraventricular Tachycardia

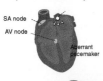

Junctional (nodal)

Definition/Recognition
Adult dog HR > 180 bpm
Adult cat HR > 240 bpm
P wave different configuration than sinus P wave
Negative P wave suggests junctional origin

Causes
Atrial dilatation from first degree cardiac disease
Elevated sympathetic tone
Ischemia
Electrolyte imbalances
Hyperthyroidism
Drugs/toxins

Treatment
Vagal maneuvers may abruptly stop the arrhythmia (helps to differentiate from sinus tachycardia)
If arrhythmia causing clinical signs:
1) digoxin; 2) diltiazem 0.25 mg/kg slow (over 20 min) IV, through peripheral vein, to effect; 3) Goal: HR to ~160-180 bpm (dog) and 200 bpm (cat) and to improve perfusion
Check CRT, mucous-membrane color, pulses, mental status q1h

C Atrial Fibrillation

Definition/Recognition
No visible P waves in any lead
Irregularly irregular rhythm
Normal QRS morphology
Rapid HR
Chaotic (variable intensity) and irregular heart sounds
Dropped pulses, weak pulses
Often poor CRT, pale mucous-membrane color, weakness

Causes
Atrial dilatation from primary degree cardiac disease
DCM-large breed canine
HCM-feline
CVD- small-breed canine

Treatment
Goal is to slow AV node conduction to ventricular response rate and improve perfusion
Digoxin
Diltiazem

D VPCs and Ventricular Tachycardia (VT)

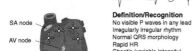

Definition/Recognition
P waves unassociated with QRS
QRS morphology is wide and bizarre
May see fusion beats or capture beats
Rhythm is rapid (VT) and regular
May see poor pulses, dropped pulses, pale cyanotic mucous membrane, poor CRT, weakness, and syncope

Causes
Primary degree cardiac disease
Systemic disease-hypoxia, hypotension, shock, sepsis, DIC, hyperthermia, hypokalemia, can worsen VT

Treatment
Generally treatment is indicated if:
1. The arrhythmia is associated with clinical signs
2. The rate is rapid > 180 bpm (dog); 240 bpm (cat)
3. Multiform VPCs present
4. R on T seen
5. CHF present
Drugs used
1. Lidocaine 4 mg/kg IV bolus (dog) and 0.4 mg/kg (cat)
2. Lidocaine CRI @ 40-80 µg/kg/min (dog); 10 µg/kg/min (cat) if lidocaine bolus worked
3. Procainamide 2-20 mg/kg IV over 20 min (dog); 1-2 mg/kg IV slow (cat), followed by CRI @ 25 µg/g/min (dog), 10 µg/kg/min (cat)
4. Propranolol 0.25-0.5 mg slow IV to effect q 5 min max 5 mg in dogs, max 0.5 mg in cats

E Ventricular Fibrillation

Definition/Recognition
Lack of defined QRS
Irregular rhythm
Low-amplitude waves of variable morphology

Causes
Primary degree cardiac disease
Systemic disease

Treatment
1. Defibrillate immediately
   External: 2 J/kg (<7kg), 5 J/kg (8-40 kg), 10 J/kg (>40 kg)
   Internal: 0.2 J/kg
2. Begin cardiocerebropulmonary resuscitation simultaneously IV fluids, colloids
3. If defibrillation successful, give lidocaine (2 mg/kg) IV to ↑ threshold for refibrillation
4. Pharmacologic defibrillation: KCl 1 mEq/kg IV, then CaCl$_2$ 10% 0.2 mL/kg IV

Premature Depolarizations and Tachyarrhythmias

These arrhythmias are commonly caused by ischemic, toxic, metabolic, inflammatory, or degenerative processes affecting the myocardium. These etiological factors induce ectopic pacemaker activity or re-entrant pathways that result in development of these arrhythmias.

Supraventricular Tachyarrhythmias

- Atrial-premature depolarizations **(Part A)**. These occur at a shorter cycle interval than the period between the normal sinus-origin depolarizations for an animal. The QRS complexes of premature atrial depolarizations are morphologically similar to those of sinus beats as conduction to the ventricles is through normal conduction pathways. The treatment of atrial premature depolarizations is directed toward the underlying cause (e.g., CHF).
- Supraventricular tachycardia (heart rate >240 bpm) **(Part B)**. One of the most important aspects with supraventricular tachycardia is to differentiate it from sinus tachycardia. The causes of sinus tachycardia should be ruled out and include dehydration, hypovolemia, hyperthermia, infection, pain, and cardiac disease (e.g., CHF). With supraventricular tachycardia, vagal maneuvers can abruptly stop the rhythm. The treatment for supraventricular tachycardia associated with normal cardiac structure and function involves administration of calcium channel blockers (diltiazem 1–2 mg/kg PO tid) or β-adrenergic blocking agents such as propranolol (1 mg/kg PO bid–tid). If supraventricular tachycardia manifests in the setting of CHF, the use of cardiac glycosides is a primary therapeutic consideration (see Atrial fibrillation).
- Atrial fibrillation **(Part C)**. On auscultation of animals with atrial fibrillation there is a chaotic (varying intensity and rhythm)-sounding heart. The rate is usually rapid and the animal may or may not be in respiratory distress. On the ECG, no P waves can be identified and the rhythm is irregularly irregular. The most common cause is atrial enlargement secondary to cardiomyopathy or other causes of CHF. The goal of therapy in small animals is to decrease the ventricular response rate (slow AV conduction). Digoxin administration (0.01 mg/kg PO divided bid) is the drug of choice to decrease conduction through the AV node in dogs. In cats, diltiazem (7.5 mg PO tid) or atenolol (6.25–12.50 mg PO once daily) administration can slow the ventricular response rate. The goal is to slow the ventricular response rate to approximately 180 bpm in dogs and 200 bpm in cats.

Ventricular Tachyarrhythmias

- Ventricular premature depolarizations and paroxysmal tachycardia **(Part D)**. Ventricular premature depolarizations typically appear wide and bizarre with respect to QRS complex morphology on ECG tracings. These depolarizations do not resemble the normal QRS complex because the impulse is generated below the AV node and conduction through the ventricles is through myocyte pathways instead of the Purkinje network. The rhythmic discharge of these impulses is often from re-entrant pathways causing local repeated depolarizations. With the development of paroxysmal or sustained ventricular tachycardia, the rapid rhythm (from the irritable or triggered ventricular focus) becomes the pacemaker of the heart. The treatment of ventricular premature depolarizations and nonsustained ventricular tachycardia involves management of the underlying disease process and administration of ventricular antiarrhythmic drugs. Animals with uniform, isolated ventricular premature depolarizations and normal cardiac structure and function may require only monitoring and no treatment unless clinical signs of syncope or weakness develop. In animals with heart disease or clinical signs attributable to frequent, multiform ventricular premature depolarizations and paroxysmal ventricular tachycardia, the administration of sustained-release procainamide (10–20 mg/kg PO tid in dogs) or the administration of atenolol (6.25–12.50 mg PO once daily in cats) is the recommended treatment.
- Sustained ventricular tachycardia (>160 bpm in dogs and >200 bpm in cats). The etiology and recognition of sustained ventricular tachycardia are as described in the section on ventricular premature depolarizations. The approach for managing patients with sustained ventricular tachycardia involves assessment for and correction of extracardiac influences on cardiac conduction such as hypovolemia, acidosis, hypokalemia, hypoxemia, hyperthermia, and pain. If the arrhythmia is causing severe hemodynamic instability or persists despite the treatment of these extracardiac factors, lidocaine administration is indicated. Initial use of lidocaine involves IV bolus administration (2 mg/kg in dogs, 0.5 mg/kg in cats). This lidocaine bolus administration can be repeated up to 3 times in 10–15 minutes to obtain conversion to normal sinus rhythm. Following successful conversion to normal sinus rhythm, lidocaine (40–80 μg/kg/min) is administered by constant-rate IV infusion in dogs and β-adrenergic blocking agent (propranolol 2.5 mg PO tid) is administered in cats to maintain antiarrhythmic effects. If lidocaine administration is not successful, a constant-rate IV infusion of procainamide (20–40 μg/kg/min) can be attempted in dogs. Continuous ECG monitoring along with serial assessment of body temperature, pulse, and respiratory parameters is required in animals with ventricular tachycardia. The use of oxygen supplementation, pain management, and appropriate therapy for electrolyte and acid-base disturbances is critical to successful antiarrhythmic treatment in these patients.
- Ventricular fibrillation **(Part E)**. Multiple areas of the ventricular muscle depolarize simultaneously, causing a loss of coordination of contraction with minimal ejection of blood and the development of cardiopulmonary arrest. This malignant arrhythmia can be initiated by progression of ventricular tachyarrhythmias associated with ischemia of the heart muscle or conduction system, electrolyte or acid-base abnormalities and drugs (anesthetic agents) or toxins, and electric shock. Initiation of ventricular fibrillation often is associated with complexes on the ECG that are relatively coarse (wider) as bundles of muscle depolarize simultaneously (limited coordination of electrical events). As ventricular fibrillation persists, the dispersion of depolarization causes smaller sections of muscle to depolarize simultaneously, resulting in fine (narrow) fibrillation complexes on the ECG. It is usually easier to defibrillate an animal with coarse fibrillation; in general, the longer fibrillation persists, the less likely defibrillation attempts will be successful.

Defibrillation requires the administration of a strong electrical current to stop the fibrillation through simultaneous, global depolarization of the ventricles. If a defibrillator is available, it is used immediately upon a diagnosis of ventricular fibrillation. The dose of current applied ranges from 5 to 10 J/kg for initial attempts at external defibrillation and from 10 to 50 J for defibrillation associated with internal cardiac massage cardiopulmonary resuscitation methods. The co-administration of epinephrine (1 mL of 1:1,000 epinephrine/5 kg IV) may aid in the successful defibrillation of the patient. If defibrillation attempts return the patient to a coordinated ECG activity that allows spontaneous circulation of blood, continuous monitoring of the ECG along with ongoing support of hemodynamics is required for successful management.

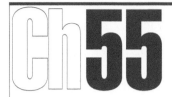

Thromboembolism

Elizabeth Rozanski

A   **Thromboembolism**

Stasis

Vascular damage

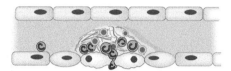

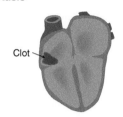

Clot

Prothrombotic Tendencies

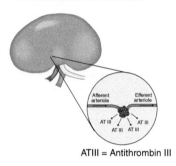

Afferent
arteriole   Efferent
arteriole

AT III   AT III
AT III   AT III

ATIII = Antithrombin III

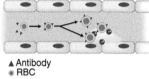

▲ Antibody
◉ RBC

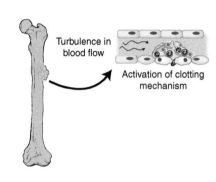

Turbulence in
blood flow

Activation of clotting
mechanism

B

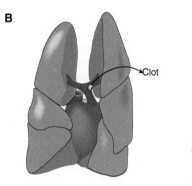

Clot

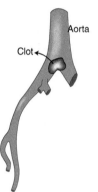

Aorta

Clot

C   **Heparin** ———→ Binding AT III ————→ Amplified inhibition of prothrombin,
factor X inside blood vessel

Coumadin ———→ Preventing synthesis of active factors (II, VII, IX, X)

D

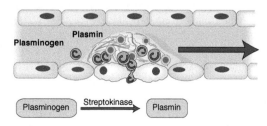

Plasmin

Plasminogen

Plasminogen	Streptokinase	Plasmin

Thromboembolic diseases are common complications in the critically ill. In the normal animal, there is a tightly controlled balance between the procoagulant and anticoagulant properties of the vascular system. Thrombi (and eventually emboli) form because of a disturbance in the balance in this system that results in a hypercoagulable state. There are 3 important factors responsible for the eventual development of thrombi (see **Part A**). These include changes in the vessel endothelium, impairment of blood flow (stasis), and development of prothrombotic tendencies in the blood. These 3 factors are referred to as *Virchow's triad*. It is important to understand that all prothrombotic tendencies may be traced to a defect in at least 1 of these 3 areas.

Risk Factors

In people, most pulmonary embolic disease is believed to arise from deep vein thrombosis (DVT). Currently the incidence of DVT in dogs is not known, but the risk factors for the development of thromboembolic disease in dogs are sepsis, neoplasia, heart disease including heartworm infection, immune-mediated hemolytic anemia, and protein-losing nephropathy or enteropathy. In cats, almost all thromboembolic disease is arterial thromboembolism. Arterial thromboembolism usually arises in cats with cardiomyopathy and an accompanying enlarged left atrium.

Clinical Signs

Clinical signs of thromboembolic disease depend on the affected organ and the size of the embolus. The magnitude of the clinical signs generally reflects the size of the clot burden (**Part B**). The most common type of thromboembolic disease detected in dogs is pulmonary thromboembolism (PTE). Clinical signs of PTE include respiratory distress in a critically ill dog. Occasionally, a loud or split S_2 sound may be auscultated owing to concurrent pulmonary hypertension. Other potential differential diagnoses include heart failure, pneumonia, and acute respiratory distress syndrome (ARDS). Venous thromboembolism in dogs may be clinically silent or associated with swelling of the limb. Signs of peripheral arterial thromboembolism reflect the location of the embolus and may include signs of CNS disturbance, myocardial infarction, or other end-organ dysfunction. Arterial thromboembolism to a limb may be associated with the five "P's"—pain, pulselessness, pallor, paresis, and poikilothermy.

Diagnosis

Diagnosis of thromboembolism may be challenging. In the circumstance of suspected PTE, chest radiographs may demonstrate blunted pulmonary arteries or regions of oligemia (decreased blood flow), or may show patchy interstitial to alveolar infiltrates, right-sided cardiac enlargement, or pleural effusion. However, normal-appearing chest radiographs do not exclude PTE. Echocardiography may document pulmonary hypertension, and occasionally a thrombus may be visualized. Ventilation-perfusion (V/Q) scans are used widely in people to attempt to document the areas of decreased ventilation. Angiography is considered the "gold standard" to document areas of decreased perfusion and may be performed to document the presence of PTE. Computed tomography (CT) has been used in people to try to document the presence of thromboembolic disease. Some of the new helical CT scanners may be able to perform an entire scan of the thorax in 30–60 seconds. This technology appears to offer some promise for some critically ill veterinary patients.

Laboratory testing occasionally provides some confirmatory evidence for PTE. Many dogs with PTE have thrombocytopenia (<120,000 platelets/μL). Arterial blood gas analysis of affected dogs classically shows hypoxemia with hypocarbia and a respiratory alkalosis. These findings are nonspecific for PTE but do help to support a diagnosis. d-Dimer analysis has been used in people with suspected PTE. d-Dimers are a specific type of fibrin-degradation product. A positive result for d-dimers suggests that PTE is possible, while a negative result appears to exclude the possibility of PTE. The utility of d-dimers in animals with suspected PTE is unknown.

Diagnosis of cats with ATE is typically based on clinical signs compatible with arterial thrombosis, although other confirmatory tests such as angiography also can be performed. Ultrasound examination of the aortic bifurcation may document the presence of a thromboembolism. A blood sample taken from the affected limb will be hypoglycemic relative to a sample from a nonaffected limb.

Therapy

Therapy for an animal with presumed thromboembolic disease is divided into specific and supportive care. In some cases, the body's own thrombolytic system will eventually dissolve the clot and restore adequate perfusion to the tissues. In general, supportive care is limited to supplemental oxygen or ventilatory therapy and intravascular fluid support. In some cases, it may be difficult to distinguish PTE from other causes of respiratory distress such as heart failure or pneumonia. In these cases, initial empirical treatment also should include therapy (e.g., antibiotics, diuretics) for the other possible conditions. Specific therapy for thromboembolic disease includes anticoagulants and fibrinolytic therapies. Therapy with anticoagulants is not effective for the existing clot but may prevent further clot formation or extension of the existing clot. Anticoagulants that may be used include Warfarin (Coumadin) and heparin (**Part C**). Warfarin administration is required for at least 2 days to reach therapeutic effect, so it is not a rational choice in animals with acute signs of thromboembolic disease. In recent years, heparin therapy has been used in animal patients considered at risk of thromboembolism (e.g., sepsis, immune-mediated hemolytic anemia). The recommended dose for heparin administration ranges from 10–15 IU/kg to 250–300 IU/kg.

Thrombolytic therapy has occasionally been used in animals with signs of thromboembolism. The thrombolytics used in veterinary patients include streptokinase (**Part D**) and tissue plasminogen activator (TPA). These fibrinolytic agents act to dissolve formed clots. The administration of thrombolytics in veterinary patients has been limited, although some results have been encouraging. For example, streptokinase administration (IV at 90,000 U in 20 minutes followed by 45,000 U hourly for 3 additional hours) has been used to successfully resolve ATE in some cats. Potential complications of the use of thrombolytics include bleeding, particularly from previous venipuncture sites, and local or systemic reperfusion injury associated with the production of oxygen radicals. Massive reoxygenation and perfusion of tissues can be observed in some cats with ATE that receive thrombolytic treatment, and result in metabolic acidosis, hyperkalemia, and a host of other metabolic disturbances.

Prevention

Prevention of thromboembolic disease is divided into recognition of the patient at risk (see **Part A**), efforts to limit risk, and anticoagulant therapy. Efforts to limit risk can include successful therapy for the underlying disease process, earlier return to mobility including physical therapy, and early removal of unnecessary IV catheters. Although protocols for prophylactic anticoagulant therapy in animals are not well established, options include heparin administration for the hospitalized patient and administration of aspirin, warfarin, or low-molecular-weight heparin for the convalescent period.

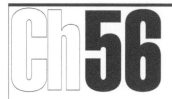

Acute Hepatic Failure: Recognition and Treatment

Robert J. Murtaugh

A   Selected Causes of Hepatic Necrosis

Chemicals
Drugs
Aflatoxin
Septicemia
Acute pancreatitis
Inflammatory bowel disease
Viral agents
Inflammatory hepatic disease
Systemic hypoxia
Anemia
Ischemic injury
Excessive copper storage
Heartworm-associated conditions (e.g. postcaval syndrome)
Trauma

B   Selected Drugs Known to Cause Hepatic Disease

Acetaminophen
Anabolic steroids
Anticonvulsant drugs
Antineoplastic drugs (methotrexate, L-asparaginase, 6-mercaptopurine
Arsenicals
Diethylcarbamazine
Furosemide
Glucocortoids
Inhalation anesthetics (halothane, methoxyflurane)
Ketoconazole
Carprofen
Mitotane (o.p.'-DDD)
Sulfonamides
Tetracycline

C   Hepatic failure

Laboratory finding:

$\uparrow$ ALT
$\uparrow$ Bilirubin
$\downarrow\uparrow$ Glucose
$\downarrow$ Clotting factors
$\uparrow$ Bile acids
$\uparrow$ Ammonia

Liver

D   Ascites

Kidney

Renin → $\uparrow$ Aldosterone

$\uparrow$ Sympathetic tone

$\uparrow$ Sodium/ water retention
$\uparrow$ Potassium excretion
$\uparrow$ Bicarbonate reabsorption

Decreased filling
$\downarrow$ Cardiac output

Heart

Hypokalemia and metabolic alkalosis

E   Hepatic failure with $\uparrow$ NH$_3$ reaching brain

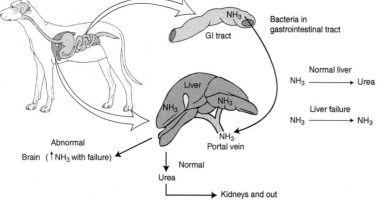

NH$_3$
GI tract

Bacteria in gastrointestinal tract

Liver

NH$_3$ NH$_3$

NH$_3$
Portal vein

Normal liver
NH$_3$ ———→ Urea

Liver failure
NH$_3$ ———→ NH$_3$

Abnormal

Brain ($\uparrow$NH$_3$ with failure)

Normal

Urea

Kidneys and out

F   Factors That Precipitate Metabolic Changes Leading to Hepatic Encephalopathy

Increased dietary protein intake
GI hemorrhage
Diuretic administration
Sedative or barbiturate administration
Uremia
Infection or Endotoxemia
Constipation
Large intestinal bacterial overgrowth
Methionine administration

G   Selected Complications of Acute Liver Failure Requiring Treatment

Anemia
Hypoglycemia
Coagulopathies
Sepsis
Ascites

Severe hepatic failure can result as an end stage of any chronic hepatopathy or as a consequence of acute hepatic necrosis. Since the hepatocyte is exposed to an extensive portal and systemic venous circulation, it is susceptible to injury by a variety of agents (**Parts A** and **B**).

Clinical Features

The clinical features of animals with acute fulminant hepatic failure range from profound depression to coma, with the degree of hepatic encephalopathy depending on the cause and severity. Vomiting, icterus, anorexia, and fever are often seen. The presence of coagulopathies such as disseminated intravascular coagulation (DIC) reflects the severity of liver damage, and they usually manifest with GI bleeding, hematemesis, ecchymoses, and excessive bleeding at venipuncture sites.

Laboratory findings may include increases in serum ALT and AST activity. The concentrations of serum alkaline phosphatase, serum γ-glutamyltransferase, serum bilirubin, serum glucose, and clotting factors are variable (**Part C**). Hepatic function tests such as measurements of serum bile acids and plasma ammonia concentration reveal the degree of hepatic failure.

Treatment

The cornerstone of treatment includes elimination of the inciting cause (such as drugs or toxins), providing optimal conditions for hepatic regeneration, preventing complications, and reversing derangements occurring with hepatic failure. The multitude of derangements occurring with acute hepatic failure relate to the many functions of the liver to maintain homeostasis.

Fluid Therapy

Patients with severe hepatic failure frequently have dehydration and hypokalemia. In addition to other deleterious effects, hypokalemia contributes greatly to the severity of hepatic encephalopathy. The most common acid-base disturbance with hepatic disease is alkalosis, although other disturbances can be seen (**Part D**). If prerenal azotemia occurs, excess urea will diffuse into the colon, where it becomes a substrate for ammonia production and thus worsens encephalopathy.

Management of these derangements requires aggressive IV fluid therapy, and the fluid of choice is best determined by measurement of serum electrolyte and arterial blood gas levels. In general, the fluid of choice is half-strength saline solution (0.45%) with 2.5% dextrose, supplemented with potassium chloride. Potassium chloride should be added at the rate of 30 mEq/L of fluids until serum potassium concentration is known, at which time the concentration administered can be adjusted. Ringer's solution or 0.9% saline solution is an acceptable alternative; however, the higher sodium content makes each less desirable because many patients with hepatic disease have excessive sodium retention and administration of either solution can exacerbate ascites. Lactated Ringer's solution should be avoided because lactate is converted to bicarbonate in the liver, and the alkalinization may exacerbate hepatoencephalopathy.

Short-Term Management of Hepatic Encephalopathy

The approach to managing acute hepatic encephalopathy involves reducing the formation and absorption of encephalopathic toxins from the intestinal tract (**Parts E** and **F**), avoiding drugs that exacerbate encephalopathy (e.g., tranquilizers, anticonvulsants, anesthetics), and controlling GI hemorrhage and other complications (**Part G**).

The therapeutic efforts designed to reduce the formation and absorption of encephalopathic toxins are directed primarily toward reducing ammonia absorption, despite the importance of other encephalopathic toxins such as mercaptans, short-chain fatty acids, and aromatic amino acids. Since ammonia is produced primarily in the colon from bacterial action on dietary amines (proteins) and urea (which diffuses from the systemic circulation into the colon), efforts at lowering the blood ammonia concentration are aimed at interrupting this process.

Large-volume (50 mL/kg body weight) cleansing enemas are used to decrease colonic bacterial numbers. The enema solution should be composed of normal saline solution with povidone-iodine added to make 1:100 solution to further decrease colonic bacterial numbers. Saline also has the advantage of lowering colonic pH trapping ammonia (NH_3) as the nonabsorbable ammonium ion. Enemas should be retained as long as possible and repeated often (up to every 2 hours) as necessary to manage the neurologic manifestations of encephalopathy and hepatic coma.

Lactulose administration is another useful adjunct to decrease ammonia absorption. Lactulose is a disaccharide that undergoes minimal absorption in the stomach and small intestine, reaching the colon unchanged. In the colon it is metabolized by bacteria, resulting in the formation of low-molecular-weight acids that acidify the colonic contents. In addition, the metabolic by-products of lactulose induce an osmotic catharsis and therefore lower colonic bacterial numbers. The initial empirical dose of lactulose is 1.0 mL/kg every 2–4 hours. The dose can be titrated to cause feces to have a soft consistency; excessive amounts of lactulose will cause diarrhea. Orally administered antibiotics (metronidazole; 6–10 mg/kg po TID) also can be helpful to decrease colonic bacterial numbers.

Avoiding Drugs That Exacerbate Encephalopathy

Drugs that depress the CNS should be avoided because of their potential to exacerbate hepatic encephalopathy. These patients have increased cerebral sensitivity to CNS depressants. In addition, drugs that are cleared by the liver have prolonged activity, owing to decreased hepatic clearance in animals with liver failure. Analgesics, tranquilizers, sedatives, anesthetics, and barbiturates should be avoided if possible. If sedation is necessary, these drugs should be used in decreased doses. Diuretics such as furosemide should be given with caution because they can exacerbate hypovolemia, prerenal azotemia, hypokalemia, metabolic alkalosis, and hepatic encephalopathy.

Controlling GI Hemorrhage

Patients with hepatic disease are prone to GI hemorrhage due to hypergastrinemia, mucosal microthrombosis, and coagulopathies. The result of GI hemorrhage is increased ammonia production. In addition, GI hemorrhage leads to hypovolemia, shock, and hypoxia. These effects also exacerbate encephalopathy. The treatment of GI hemorrhage involves specific therapy with drugs that inhibit gastric acid secretion such as ranitidine or omeprazole.

Nutritional Management

Nutritional management of hepatic failure should include the following considerations: 1) Calories from protein should be moderately restricted, and for enteral nutrition, ingredients that are of high biological value and highly digestible should be fed in small, frequent amounts. Cottage cheese is an ideal protein source. 2) Protein sources with high branched-chain acid to aromatic amino acid ratios are preferred for parenteral nutrition. 3) Carbohydrates should supply most nonprotein calories. 4) Sodium and copper intake should be restricted. 5) Supplementation with zinc, ascorbic acid, and a salt and copper-free vitamin-mineral may be helpful.

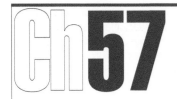

Acute Pancreatitis I: Pathophysiology and Diagnosis

Alison R. Gaynor

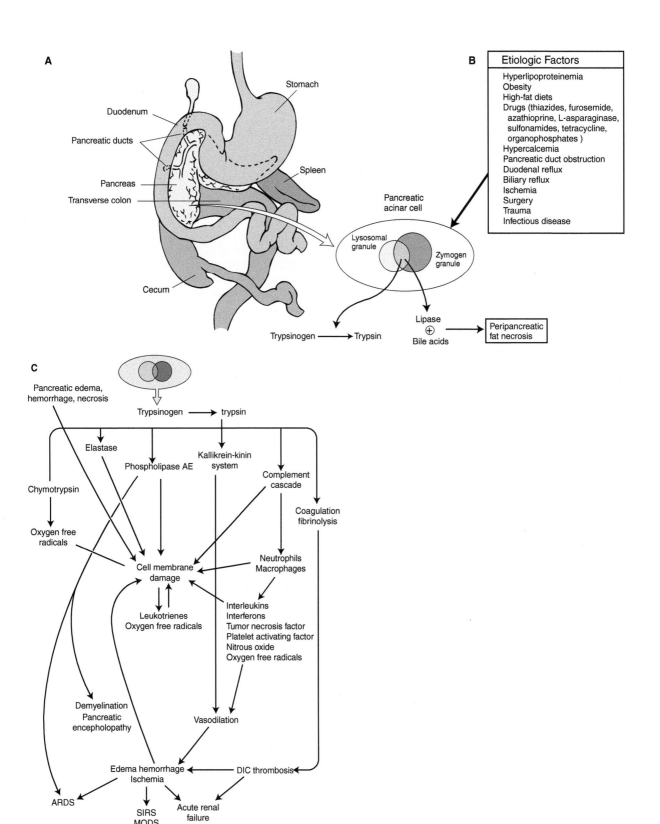

A

Stomach

Duodenum

Pancreatic ducts

Pancreas

Transverse colon

Cecum

Spleen

Pancreatic acinar cell

Lysosomal granule

Zymogen granule

Trypsinogen → Trypsin

Lipase ⊕ Bile acids → Peripancreatic fat necrosis

B

Etiologic Factors
Hyperlipoproteinemia
Obesity
High-fat diets
Drugs (thiazides, furosemide, azathioprine, L-asparaginase, sulfonamides, tetracycline, organophosphates)
Hypercalcemia
Pancreatic duct obstruction
Duodenal reflux
Biliary reflux
Ischemia
Surgery
Trauma
Infectious disease

C

Pancreatic edema, hemorrhage, necrosis

Trypsinogen → trypsin

Elastase

Chymotrypsin

Phospholipase AE

Kallikrein-kinin system

Complement cascade

Coagulation fibrinolysis

Oxygen free radicals

Cell membrane damage

Neutrophils Macrophages

Leukotrienes Oxygen free radicals

Interleukins
Interferons
Tumor necrosis factor
Platelet activating factor
Nitrous oxide
Oxygen free radicals

Demyelination Pancreatic encepholopathy

Vasodilation

Edema hemorrhage Ischemia

DIC thrombosis

ARDS

SIRS MODS

Acute renal failure

Pancreatitis, broadly classified as acute, recurrent, or chronic, is a fairly common disease in dogs and is becoming more widely recognized in cats. Acute pancreatitis and recurrent acute pancreatitis are characterized by episodes of pancreatic inflammation with a sudden onset and few or no permanent clinical or pathologic, changes. Episodes may range in severity from mild and self-limiting to severe fulminant disease with extensive necrosis, systemic inflammation or sepsis, and multiorgan failure. Local complications such as infected pancreatic necrosis, pancreatic pseudocysts, and pancreatic abscesses also may occur.

Pathophysiology

A number of factors have been implicated as potential causes of pancreatitis (**Parts A** and **B**). Most cases in dogs and cats, however, are considered to be idiopathic, since a direct causal relationship is infrequently demonstrated. Furthermore, the mechanisms by which these various factors cause pancreatitis and their significance in naturally occurring disease remain speculative. Regardless of the underlying etiology, acute pancreatitis involves intrapancreatic activation of digestive enzymes with resultant pancreatic autodigestion. Studies of animal models suggest that this occurs within the acinar cell by abnormal fusion of normally segregated lysosomes with zymogen granules (catalytically inactive forms of pancreatic enzymes), resulting in premature activation of trypsinogen to trypsin (see **Part B**). Trypsin in turn activates other proenzymes, setting in motion a cascade of local and systemic effects that are responsible for the clinical signs of acute pancreatitis.

In the normal animal, several defense systems exist to discourage pancreatic autodigestion. These include segregation of pancreatic enzymes from the rest of the cytosol from the time of synthesis, and synthesis, storage, and secretion of most pancreatic enzymes as inactive proenzymes (zymogens), which become activated after cleavage of an activation peptide at the amino terminus. In addition, a specific trypsin inhibitor (pancreatic specific trypsin inhibitor) is synthesized, stored, and co-secreted with the digestive enzymes, presumably to immediately inactivate any small amounts of trypsin formed prior to secretion in the duodenum. Circulating plasma protease inhibitors, α_1-protease inhibitor (α_1-antitrypsin) and particularly α_2-macroglobulin, are vital in protecting against the effects of proteases in the vascular space. Proteases bound to α_2-macroglobulin retain some catalytic activity, but these complexes are cleared rapidly by the monocyte-macrophage system. When all of these protective mechanisms are overwhelmed, local and systemic manifestations of pancreatitis develop (**Part C**). Subsequent to inappropriate activation of trypsin, further activation of all zymogens, particularly proelastase and prophospholipase A_2, will amplify pancreatic and peripancreatic damage and may transform mild edematous pancreatic inflammation to hemorrhagic or necrotic pancreatitis. Local ischemia, phospholipase A_2, and oxygen free radicals, produced in part from activation of xanthine oxidase by chymotrypsin, disrupt cell membranes, leading to pancreatic hemorrhage and necrosis, increased capillary permeability, and initiation of the arachidonic acid cascade. Elastase also causes increased vascular permeability secondary to degradation of elastin in vessel walls. Phospholipase A_2 degrades surfactant, thus promoting development of pulmonary edema and the adult respiratory distress syndrome (ARDS). Trypsin may activate the complement cascade, leading to an influx of inflammatory cells and production of multiple cytokines and more free radicals. Trypsin can also activate

the kallikrein-kinin system, resulting in vasodilation, hypotension, and possibly acute renal failure, and the coagulation and fibrinolytic pathways, resulting in microvascular thromboses and disseminated intravascular coagulation (DIC).

Clinical Presentation

Acute pancreatitis seems to occur more frequently in middle-aged and older dogs and may be more common in those that are overweight; have a history of prior or recurrent GI disturbances; or have diabetes mellitus, hypothyroidism, or hyperadrenocorticism. Dogs with acute pancreatitis usually are presented because of anorexia, vomiting, depression, and sometimes diarrhea. They may be febrile and often exhibit signs of abdominal discomfort. Common clinical signs in cats with acute pancreatitis include lethargy, anorexia, dehydration, and hypothermia; vomiting and abdominal pain are reported less frequently. With severe acute pancreatitis in either species, signs of systemic complications including dyspnea, icterus, bleeding disorders, cardiac arrhythmias, oliguria, shock, and collapse.

Diagnosis

Diagnosis of acute pancreatitis requires careful integration of historical, physical examination, laboratory, and diagnostic imaging findings combined with a high degree of suspicion. Neutrophilic leukocytosis is common, as is an elevated hematocrit reflecting dehydration, although anemia also may be seen, especially in cats. Elevations in hepatic enzyme activities and total bilirubin are often noted. Animals are frequently azotemic, usually from prerenal causes, although acute renal failure may also be present. Hyperglycemia is common and is thought to be secondary to stress-related increases. Hypoglycemia may be seen if systemic inflammation or sepsis are present. Mild to moderate hypocalcemia and hypomagnesemia are often reported, possibly as a result of pancreatic and peripancreatic fat saponification. Other common findings include hypoalbuminemia secondary to GI losses and sequestration, and hypercholesterolemia and hypertriglyceridemia. Increased activities of lipase and amylase historically have been used as markers of pancreatitis, but are of limited diagnostic value because elevations also may occur from extrapancreatic sources such as azotemia and glucocorticoid administration. Furthermore, lipase and amylase activities are often within normal limits in animals with confirmed pancreatitis, particularly cats. Elevations in trypsin-like immunoreactivity may suggest a diagnosis of pancreatitis, but also occur with azotemia.

Abdominal radiographs may provide supportive evidence and are especially valuable in helping to rule out other causes of an acute abdomen such as intestinal obstruction or perforation. Common radiographic signs include increased density and loss of detail ("ground glass") in the right cranial abdomen, and displacement of the descending duodenum to the right with widening of the angle between the proximal duodenum and the pylorus. Abdominal ultrasonography is particularly helpful both as a diagnostic tool. The pancreas may appear enlarged and hypoechoic, and masses, localized inflammation, and focal fluid accumulations may be identified. Detection of amylase and lipase activities in fluid obtained by diagnostic peritoneal lavage that are higher than those in serum strongly suggests a diagnosis of pancreatitis. Cytologic examination of abdominal fluid may aid in detecting local complications such as infected necrosis, which may require surgical intervention.

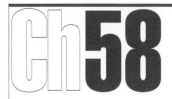

Acute Pancreatitis II: Treatment

Alison R. Gaynor

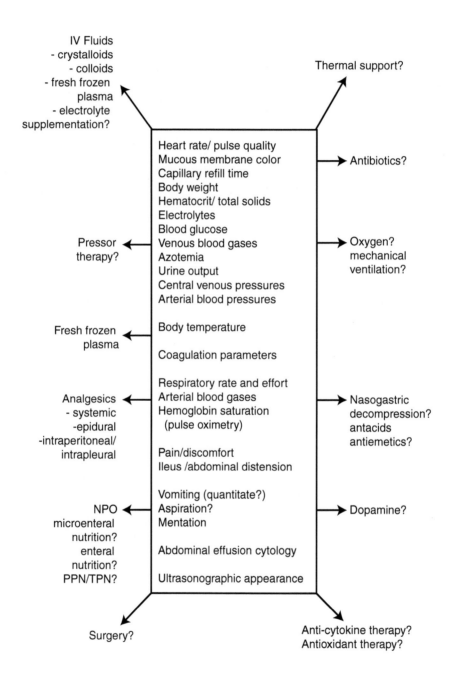

IV Fluids
- crystalloids
- colloids
- fresh frozen
  plasma
- electrolyte
supplementation?

Thermal support?

Antibiotics?

Pressor
therapy?

Oxygen?
mechanical
ventilation?

Heart rate/ pulse quality
Mucous membrane color
Capillary refill time
Body weight
Hematocrit/ total solids
Electrolytes
Blood glucose
Venous blood gases
Azotemia
Urine output
Central venous pressures
Arterial blood pressures

Body temperature

Coagulation parameters

Respiratory rate and effort
Arterial blood gases
Hemoglobin saturation
 (pulse oximetry)

Pain/discomfort
Ileus /abdominal distension

Vomiting (quantitate?)
Aspiration?
Mentation

Abdominal effusion cytology

Ultrasonographic appearance

Fresh frozen
plasma

Analgesics
- systemic
-epidural
-intraperitoneal/
intrapleural

NPO
microenteral
nutrition?
enteral
nutrition?
PPN/TPN?

Nasogastric
decompression?
antacids
antiemetics?

Dopamine?

Surgery?

Anti-cytokine therapy?
Antioxidant therapy?

Pancreatitis, broadly classified as acute, recurrent, or chronic, is a fairly common disease in dogs and is becoming more widely recognized in cats. Acute pancreatitis and recurrent acute pancreatitis are characterized by episodes of pancreatic inflammation with a sudden onset and few or no permanent clinical or pathologic, changes. Episodes may range in severity from mild and self-limiting to severe fulminant disease with extensive necrosis, systemic inflammation or sepsis, and multiorgan failure. Local complications such as infected pancreatic necrosis, pancreatic pseudocysts, and pancreatic abscesses also may occur.

Treatment

Therapy for animals with acute pancreatitis involves eliminating any identifiable underlying cause if possible, symptomatic and supportive therapy, and anticipation of and early aggressive intervention against systemic complications (**Figure**). Animals with severe disease may be hemodynamically unstable and in need of rapid resuscitation with shock-rate replacement fluids. Maintenance fluid requirement also may be substantial to combat massive ongoing fluid losses from the vascular space due to vomiting and third-spacing into the peritoneal cavity, GI tract, and the interstitium. Balanced electrolyte solutions such as lactated Ringer's are appropriate for maintenance needs but should be modified based on careful evaluation of electrolyte and acid-base status. Potassium supplementation is usually necessary. Calcium should not be supplemented unless clinical signs of tetany are observed, because of the potential for exacerbation of free radical production and cellular injury. Concurrent use of colloids such as hetastarch will reduce the volume of crystalloids needed and may help maintain intravascular volume and microcirculatory flow and reduce the degree of fluid extravasation. Use of fresh-frozen plasma is important in providing a source of albumin for oncotic pressure, clotting factors for the management of DIC, and especially a source of α_2-macroglobulins. In experimental canine pancreatitis, depletion of α_2-macroglobulins is followed rapidly by DIC, shock, and death. Frequent monitoring of blood pressure and central venous pressures as well as urine output (which may necessitate aseptic urethral catheterization with a closed collection system) may help guide rates and types of IV. fluids. Other parameters that require frequent evaluation include hematocrit and total plasma solids, blood glucose, arterial blood gases to monitor oxygenation and ventilatory status, vital signs, coagulation status renal function, and mentation. Although uncommon, persistent hyperglycemia may require insulin therapy. Analgesic therapy with systemic opioids is critical in maintaining patient comfort. Epidural and intraperitoneal analgesia are also effective, particularly in dogs. Use of antibiotics is controversial and is not recommended for mild acute pancreatitis because of the risk of inducing resistant bacterial strains. In severe cases with systemic involvement, however, judicious use of broad-spectrum antibiotics is warranted because of the high risk of bacterial translocation from the GI tract. Most deaths in human acute pancreatitis are due to septic complications. Dopamine has been shown to reduce the degree of pancreatic inflammation in experimental feline models by decreasing microvascular permeability, and may do the same in spontaneous disease. Other therapies that do not necessarily influence the outcome of acute pancreatitis but do provide patient comfort include the use of antiemetics, antacids, and nasogastric decompression.

A traditional aspect of therapy for acute pancreatitis involves withholding food and water to reduce pancreatic secretion and allow the pancreas time to recover. Most mild cases of acute pancreatitis resolve after restricting oral intake for 2–4 days, followed by gradual reintroduction of water and then small, carbohydrate-rich meals. Nutritional support is needed in severe cases in which longer periods of fasting are anticipated. Enteral feeding through a jejunostomy tube is preferred because this will help avoid mucosal atrophy and bacterial translocation, but necessitates general anesthesia and surgery. For animals that are unstable or in which surgery is not anticipated, total parenteral nutrition should be instituted. Adjunctive microenteral feeding also has been recommended, as well as nasoesophageal or gastrostomy tube feeding in cats with concurrent hepatic lipidosis that are not vomiting. If evidence of infection is detected, surgical intervention is required to debride necrotic and purulent tissue and to lavage the abdomen. Surgery also may be indicated in animals that continue to deteriorate despite aggressive medical therapy.

The Future

Diagnostic imaging modalities such as CT, dynamic contrast-enhanced CT, endoscopic retrograde cholangiopancreatography, and endoscopic ultrasonography are used routinely in human medicine and hopefully will become more widely used in veterinary medicine. Use of serum markers for diagnosis and early prediction of severity of acute pancreatitis in humans such as trypsinogen activation peptides, trypsin-α_1 protease inhibitor complexes, and cytokine levels (IL-6 and IL-8) are not currently available in veterinary species but is under investigation. Specific therapies using direct inhibitors of pancreatic secretion (atropine, somatostatin, glucagon, calcitonin) or using protease and other pancreatic enzyme inhibitors generally have proved unsuccessful. However, with increasing recognition of the importance of inflammatory mediators in the progression to systemic organ dysfunction, recent studies into the use of free radical scavengers and cytokine antagonists, particularly platelet-activating factor antagonists, are showing promising results.

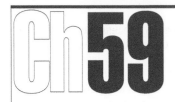

Diabetic Ketoacidosis

Nancy S. Taylor

A. Heterogenic Causes of Diabetes Mellitus in Animals

Genetic predisposition
Pancreatic injury
  Trauma
  Neoplasia
  Infection
  Autoantibodies
  Inflammation
  Drugs
Hormone-induced β-cell exhaustion
  Growth hormone
  Thyroid hormones
  Cortisol
  Catecholamines
  Progestins
Target tissue insensitivity
  Decreased number of insulin receptors
  Defective insulin receptors
  Defect in postreceptor effects
Dyshormonogenesis of insulin

B. Combined effects of acute insulin withdrawal

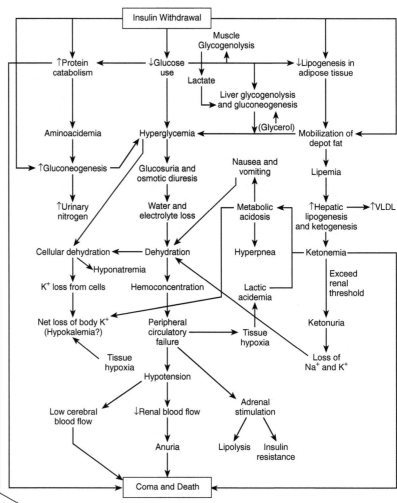

C.

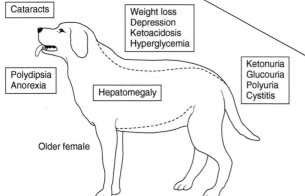

Diabetic ketoacidosis (DKA) is a serious complication of diabetes mellitus (DM) and carries a high mortality if it is managed improperly. For DKA to occur there has to be a relative or absolute deficiency of insulin combined with increased diabetogenic (stress) hormones, which results in dehydration, hypovolemia, metabolic acidosis (lactic and ketoacids), and electrolyte abnormalities (**Parts A** and **B**).

Diagnosis

Clinical signs of diabetes include polyuria, polydipsia, polyphagia, and weight loss. The diagnosis of DM is based on persistent hyperglycemia and glucosuria in a fasted animal. Ketonuria and metabolic acidosis in combination with a diagnosis of DM establish the diagnosis of DKA. At presentation the animal may be lethargic, weak, and anorexic, with vomiting and diarrhea. A fruity (ketone) smell to the breath may be noted.

Three types of ketones are produced (acetoacetone, acetone, and β-hydroxybutyrate) during anaerobic metabolism. Normal urine reagent dipsticks (Keto Diastix, Miles Lab, Elkhurt, IN) cannot detect β-hydroxybutyrate.

Calculation of the anion gap $[(Na^+ + K^+) - (Cl^- + HCO_3^-)]$ can also be helpful in the diagnosis of DKA. An anion gap >20 indicates an excess of unmeasured anions (ketoacids) is contributing to the acidemia in these animals.

Treatment

The goals are to 1) identify and treat the underlying disease process or stress factors that are contributing to the release of stress hormones or promoting insulin resistance and ketone production; 2) reduce serum glucose levels, which will halt osmotic diuresis and lower serum osmolality; 3) replace fluid lost; 4) replace electrolytes lost; and 5) restore acid-base balance (**Part C**).

Identification of Underlying Disease

To define underlying diseases or other factors that may play a role in causing DKA such as pyelonephritis, pancreatitis, pyometra, hyperadrenocorticism, urinary tract infections, renal failure, sepsis, and heart failure, an appropriate initial data base utilizing laboratory and imaging studies is required.

Replacement of Fluid Deficiencies

The provision of IV fluids is important in the reversal of dehydration. IV crystalloid fluid administration will lower plasma glucose levels by increasing glomerular filtration and urine flow. This treatment also will aid in reducing diabetogenic hormones. However, fluid treatment alone will not inhibit ketone production in the absence of insulin.

Sodium chloride (0.9% NaCl) solution is usually the IV fluid of choice unless measured serum electrolyte values indicate other choices. The patient's degree of dehydration, maintenance fluid needs, and ongoing losses (vomiting and diarrhea) should be assessed and any underlying disease that might limit the fluid administration rate (cardiac disease) should be determined. Replacement of fluid deficits should be gradual over 24–36 hours unless the patient is in shock. Hypotonic fluids should be avoided as a rapid decrease in serum osmolality may predispose to cerebral edema.

Electrolyte Replacement

As insulin treatment is initiated, serum potassium levels often fall farther as potassium shifts into cells. Life-threatening hypokalemia can occur if potassium supplementation is not provided. Potassium supplementation should be based on serum concentration (Chapter 3). Serial monitoring of serum electrolytes should be done at least twice daily in DKA patients.

As DKA is corrected, phosphorus will shift into the cells and life-threatening hypophosphatemia can occur (Chapter 10). Serum phosphorus concentrations should be monitored every 12 hours and supplementation continued until the serum phosphorus level is 2.5 mg/dL.

Insulin Therapy

Insulin is necessary to inhibit gluconeogenesis, promote glucose uptake by cells, and inhibit lipolysis and ketone production.

Regular crystalline insulin (RI) is the insulin of choice for treatment of the DKA patient until ketone production ceases and the animal is eating and drinking. RI should be administered by the IV or intramuscular (IM) route in DKA patients.

To reduce the risk of rapid fluid shifts between body fluid compartments that could result in severe electrolyte abnormalities or the development of cerebral edema, blood glucose concentrations should be lowered slowly over 6–12 hours. Ideally, blood glucose concentrations should remain >250 mg/dL for the initial 4–6 hours of insulin therapy.

For the intramuscular protocol, initially, 0.2 U of RI/kg is administered IM. RI is then administered hourly at a dose of 0.1 U/kg until the blood glucose level falls to ≤250 mg/dL. If blood glucose levels cannot be determined hourly, then the insulin should be administered every 2–4 hours during this initial treatment approach.

After the glucose level reaches 250 mg/dL, RI should be administered every 4–6 hours, with frequency and dose dependent on the serial measurement of serum glucose concentrations. When blood glucose concentration decreases to <200 mg/dL, dextrose is added to the IV fluids at a 2.5% or 5.0% concentration. Dextrose is added to the fluids in order to allow continued administration of insulin to inhibit ketone production. Insulin administration is maintained unless the blood glucose concentration decreases to <100 mg/dL.

IV infusion of RI in 0.9% saline through a continuous infusion pump is usually safe and effective for treating DKA in cats and dogs. Frequent monitoring of blood glucose concentrations is required when using this method. The initial rate for RI infusion is 1 U/kg/24 hours for dogs and 0.5 U/kg/24 hours in cats. Since insulin tends to bind to plastic tubing, 50 mL of the insulin solution should be run through the IV tubing and discarded before it is attached to the patient. When glucose levels fall to <200 mg/dL, supplementation with 2.5%–5.0% dextrose should be initiated and insulin therapy adjusted as necessary.

Restoring Acid-Base Balance

Metabolic acidosis in DKA is a result of the accumulation of ketoacids from insulin deficiency and lactic acid from hypoperfusion with a resultant exhaustion of the body's buffer system.

Correction of the acidosis in DKA patients with sodium bicarbonate administration is controversial. Treatment with insulin and IV fluids is often enough to correct the acidosis. Bicarbonate therapy is definitely indicated if the blood pH is <7.10 or the plasma bicarbonate level falls to <10 mEq/L (Chapter 16). Sodium bicarbonate administration may be warranted with less severe acidosis if the patient remains compromised following initiation of treatment with RI and improvement of tissue perfusion with IV fluid administration.

Questions

1. Which of the following statements regarding sodium re-absorption in the kidney is true?

    (A) Most of the sodium is reabsorbed in the loop of Henle
    (B) Angiotensin II directly causes sodium reabsorption from the collecting ducts
    (C) Sodium reabsorption within the nephron is always an active process
    (D) Aldosterone increases sodium reabsorption in the distal convoluted tubule by increasing the number and activity of sodium channels
    (E) Endotoxin enhances the activity of the Na^+, K^+-ATPase pump within the renal tubule cells

2. Which of the following statements regarding hypernatremia is true?

    (A) Midbrain lesions cause decreased thirst and can result in hypernatremia
    (B) The degree of hypernatremia rather than the rapidity of onset of hypernatremia has more of an effect on the patient's clinical signs
    (C) All patients with hypernatremia should be treated with rapid IV administration of 5% dextrose in water, to correct the electrolyte imbalance as quickly as possible
    (D) Hypernatremia induces the formation of idiogenic osmoles within brain cells in 3–5 days

3. Hypokalemia is commonly associated with:

    (A) Vomiting and diarrhea
    (B) Cardiac bradyarrhythmias
    (C) Hypertonic muscle tone
    (D) Metabolic acidosis
    (E) Urethral obstruction

4. If the patient's serum potassium level is 3.1 mEq/L what amount of potassium chloride should be added to each liter of maintenance fluids?

    (A) 20 mEq/L
    (B) 30 mEq/L
    (C) 40 mEq/L
    (D) 50 mEq/L
    (E) 60 mEq/L

5. Which of the following is true with regard to subcutaneous fluid administration?

    (A) All forms of crystalloid fluids can be administered subcutaneously
    (B) Up to 60 ml of fluid/kg can be administered subcutaneously in any one site
    (C) Subcutaneous fluids should be used to rehydrate a mildly dehydrated dog with a severe, superficial pyoderma
    (D) Severely dehydrated patients should be given subcutaneous fluids prior to attempting to place an IV catheter
    (E) None of the above

6. Which of the following is most true with regard to IV fluid use?

    (A) The calculation of a shock dose of IV fluids is the same, regardless of species
    (B) Maintenance fluids have a higher potassium and a lower sodium content than replacement fluids
    (C) Two-thirds of the crystalloid fluid dose remains in the vasculature an hour after administration
    (D) Shock victims should be given repeated shock doses of crystalloid fluids until their condition stabilizes
    (E) Selection of fluid type for IV administration should be based on clinician's preference

7. Which of the following is correct?

    (A) Calcium has negative inotropic and positive chronotropic effects on the heart
    (B) Furosemide causes renal calcium excretion in the proximal convoluted tubule
    (C) Acidosis cause a shift in total calcium from the ionized form to protein-bound forms
    (D) Hypercalcemia causes renal tubular ischemia and renal mineralization
    (E) Sepsis and the systemic inflammatory response syndrome are associated with hypercalcemia

8. Which of the following is true?

    (A) Hypocalcemia in patients with eclampsia can be prevented by supplementing calcium during gestation
    (B) Volume contraction is consistently associated with hypercalcemia
    (C) Primary hyperparathyroidism is the most common cause of hypercalcemia in veterinary medicine
    (D) When treating hypocalcemia, clinicians should aim for a calcium level slightly higher than normal, to prevent recurrence of clinical signs
    (E) Corticosteroids are an important component of therapy for hypercalcemia of any cause

9. Which of the following is correct?

    (A) Phosphate is the major intracellular cation
    (B) Animals with diabetic ketoacidosis that have normal or elevated serum phosphorus concentrations are not at risk for developing hypophosphatemia after receiving insulin
    (C) Increases in serum phosphorus concentration lead to parallel increases in serum ionized calcium concentration
    (D) Hypovitaminosis D may cause hypophosphatemia in part through interactions with calcium and parathyroid hormone
    (E) Metabolic acidosis causes phosphate to shift intracellularly

10. Which of the following is true?

    (A) Calcitriol is the primary regulatory hormone for renal phosphate handling

(B) Respiratory alkalosis may cause hypophosphatemia by stimulating glycolysis

(C) Serum phosphorus concentration is an accurate reflection of total-body phosphorus status

(D) Hypophosphatemia can cause decreased oxygen delivery to peripheral tissues because of diminished erythrocyte ATP concentrations

(E) IV phosphate can be safely administered in calcium-containing solutions

11. **Which of the following statements concerning hypomagnesemia is correct?**

(A) The hypokalemia associated with hypomagnesemia usually responds to replacement therapy with potassium

(B) Hypomagnesemia is readily diagnosed on the basis of low serum magnesium levels

(C) Renal magnesium losses occurring at the glomerulus play a key role in the development of hypomagnesemia

(D) Hypomagnesemia in diabetic ketoacidosis may result from osmotic diuresis, transcellular shifts, and therapeutic interventions

(E) Magnesium deficiency may predispose animals to ventricular arrhythmias by causing an increase in the ratio of intracellular to extracellular potassium

12. **Which of the following statements about hypermagnesemia is correct?**

(A) Hypermagnesemia causes increased neuromuscular excitability and ventricular tachycardia

(B) Overzealous use of cathartics in the emergency treatment of toxicoses may cause hypermagnesemia

(C) Most patients with hypermagnesemia have normal renal function

(D) Therapy for patients with severe hypermagnesemia may include mechanical ventilation and parasympatholytic agents

(E) Hypokalemia, hypocalcemia, and hyponatremia are commonly associated with hypermagnesemia

13. **Which of the following statements is most true with respect to synthetic colloids?**

(A) Hydroxyethyl starch is more effective than dextran 70 in enhancing colloidal osmotic pressure

(B) Synthetic colloids are dosed at 4 times the dose used for isotonic crystalloids

(C) Colloid infusion promotes the action of hemostatic factors and results in hypercoagulation in patients

(D) Synthetic colloids are recommended for resuscitation when the total serum solid concentrations are <3.5 gm/dL

14. **Which of the following statements is most true with respect to the hemoglobin-based oxygen carrier Oxyglobin?**

(A) The colloid osmotic pressure of Oxyglobin is greater than that of hydroxyethyl starch

(B) The P_{50} of Oxyglobin is less than that of red blood cell hemoglobin

(C) The oxyhemoglobin dissociation curve is shifted leftward for Oxyglobin compared to native hemoglobin

(D) Blood-typing and crossmatching are not required in patients prior to Oxyglobin administration

15. **Based on these results of an arterial blood gas analysis— pH 7.21, PCO_2 64 mm Hg, PO_2 69 mm Hg, HCO_3^- 25.5 mEq/L, base excess −3.1 mmol/L—what is the acid = base disturbance?**

(A) Metabolic acidosis with respiratory compensatory response, hypoxemia present

(B) Respiratory acidosis with metabolic compensatory response, hypoxemia present

(C) Metabolic alkalosis with no respiratory response

(D) Respiratory alkalosis with metabolic compensatory response

16. **Based on these results of a venous blood gas analysis— pH 7.01, PCO_2 54 mm Hg, PO_2 43 mm Hg, HCO_3^- 11 mEq/L, base excess −21 mmol/L—what is the acid-base disturbance?**

(A) Metabolic acidosis with respiratory compensation, hypoxemia present

(B) Respiratory acidosis with metabolic compensation, unable to determine oxygen status

(C) Metabolic alkalosis, respiratory acidosis, hypoxemia present

(D) Metabolic acidosis, respiratory acidosis, unable to determine oxygen status

17. **What are potential complications of $NaHCO_3$ therapy?**

(A) Hypokalemia, hypocalcemia, volume overload

(B) Hyperkalemia, paradoxical CSF acidosis, hypernatremia

(C) Iatrogenic alkalosis, hypokalemia, paradoxical CSF alkalosis

(D) Hyponatremia, volume overload, hypocalcemia

18. **How much bicarbonate should be administered to a 20-kg dog with the following blood gas values—pH 7.07 (normal 7.36–7.44), PCO_2 32.3 mm Hg (normal 36–44), HCO_3^- 9.0 mEq (normal 18–22)?**

(A) 220 mEq

(B) 66 mEq

(C) 33 mEq

(D) None

19. **Which is not a cause of respiratory acidosis?**

(A) Aspirin toxicity

(B) Pyothorax

(C) Morphine

(D) Fluid overload

20. **In a patient with chronic respiratory acidosis, what is a proper course of therapy?**

(A) Aggressive supplemental oxygen since these patients are usually hypoxemic

(B) Administration of $NaHCO_3$

(C) Fluid therapy with adequate amounts of Cl^-

(D) Aggressive ventilator therapy to bring the PCO_2 back to normal

21. **A Labrador retriever puppy is presented with a complaint of vomiting for 4 days. A gastric foreign body is diagnosed. A blood gas analysis reveals a compensated metabolic alkalosis. What therapy is needed to resolve the metabolic alkalosis?**

(A) Surgery or endoscopy to remove the foreign body
(B) Correction of volume depletion with a replacement fluid such as normal saline solution, Ringer's solution, or Normosol®
(C) Supplementation of fluids with appropriate amounts of potassium chloride
(D) All of the above

22. **A geriatric Yorkshire terrier presents in respiratory distress. A radiograph reveals a diffuse interstitial pattern. An arterial blood gas analysis reveals these values: pH 7.57, PCO_2 18 mm Hg, HCO_3^- 18 mmol/L, PO_2 54 mm Hg. What is the primary acid-base disturbance and how should the disturbance be treated?**

(A) Metabolic alkalosis; provide chloride-containing IV fluids and potassium supplementation
(B) Respiratory alkalosis; provide oxygen supplementation, since correcting hypoxemia should help resolve the hypoxemia and thus the drive to hyperventilate
(C) Respiratory alkalosis; provide oxygen supplementation, give IV HCO_3^- to increase the amount of carbon dioxide in the blood
(D) Metabolic alkalosis; provide oxygen supplementation, chloride-containing IV fluids, and potassium supplementation

23. **Which of the following conditions causing tissue hypoxia will not respond to supplemental oxygen administration?**

(A) Hypoventilation
(B) Diffusion impairment
(C) V/Q mismatch
(D) Right-to-left intrapulmonary shunt
(E) Decreased cardiac output

24. **Which of the following approaches is best with respect to administration of oxygen therapy to minimize the development of oxygen toxicity?**

(A) Keep FIO_2 between 0.4 and 0.5
(B) Keep FIO_2 between 0.5 and 0.6
(C) Minimize use of PEEP
(D) Keep PaO_2 between 80 and 90 mm Hg
(E) Keep PaO_2 between 90 and 100 mm Hg

25. **The preferred anticoagulant for use in blood stored for later transfusion is:**

(A) Heparin
(B) EDTA
(C) ACD
(D) CPDA
(E) Warfarin

26. **Cryoprecipitate:**

(A) Is prepared from fresh whole blood
(B) Is a large-volume component of fresh-frozen plasma
(C) Is rich in factor VIII activity

(D) Must be used immediately after preparation
(E) Is the preferred product to treat thrombocytopenia

27. **What are some of the "dynamic" elements in the nociceptive pathway that allow it to "rewire" itself in response to prolonged painful stimuli? (Choose all that apply.)**

(A) The recruitment of silent nociceptors
(B) Nociceptor sensitization
(C) Spinothalamic pathway
(D) WDRN windup
(E) Motivational-affective response

28. **Which area(s) of the nociceptive process allow(s) us to exert an influence to control pain generation and perception?**

(A) Suppression of the inflammatory response with NSAIDs
(B) Blockage of afferent fiber conduction with local anesthetics
(C) Targeting of opioid receptors in areas of the brain, dorsal horn, and peripherally to modulate nociceptive input
(D) All of the above

29. **Techniques that contribute to preemptive analgesia and limit postoperative pain include all of the following except:**

(A) Systemic opioids administered preoperatively
(B) Epidural opioid administration
(C) General anesthesia with inhalant gas
(D) Local anesthesia (nerve blocks)
(E) NSAIDs

30. **Epidural Analgesia is indicated for all of the following procedures except:**

(A) Hind-limb amputation in a geriatric dog with renal insufficiency
(B) Repair of fractured ileum and sacrum in a dog
(C) Femoral fracture repair in a dog with pulmonary contusions and bullae
(D) Perianal mass removal in a dog with hepatic insufficiency
(E) Treatment of severe bite wounds over the dorsal lumbar region
(F) B and E

31. **The analgesic drugs that work via activation of G proteins on cell membranes of neurons, and subsequent ion channel regulation are:**

(A) Opioids
(B) Local anesthetics
(C) α_2 Agonists
(D) Dissociative cyclohexamine anesthetics
(E) A and C

32. **Epidural anesthetic administration that migrates too far cranially after administration may result in which of the following complications?**

(A) Hypovolemia
(B) Hypotension
(C) Tachypnea
(D) Diaphragmatic flutter
(E) Forelimb rigidity

33. **Which of the following is most correct with respect to synchronous intermittent mandatory ventilation (SIMV)?**

(A) Patient can override the preset rate of breaths per minute by generating negative inspiratory pressure
(B) This mode is useful in weaning the patient from ventilatory support by decreasing the rate of breaths per minute delivered
(C) The ventilator delivers inspired gases until a preset tidal volume is achieved with each breath
(D) Pressure alarms are set to detect sudden increases in airway pressures that indicate obstruction of the tube

34. **Which of the following statements is most correct with respect to issues associated with mechanical ventilation?**

(A) PEEP is applied when blood gas analysis reveals high $PaCO_2$ concentrations
(B) Pneumothorax is a common cause of oxygen desaturation in ventilator patients
(C) Pneumonia develops less frequently in ventilator patients on antibiotics
(D) Positive-pressure ventilatory support enhances venous return to the heart

35. **Which of the following hormones is least involved in the neuroendocrine response to traumatic injury?**

(A) ACTH
(B) ADH
(C) Cortisol
(D) Epinephrine
(E) Insulin

36. **Which of the following statements concerning interventions to mediate the neuroendocrine response to traumatic injury is most correct?**

(A) Glucocorticoid support is indicated in animals with traumatic injury
(B) Crystalloid fluid administration should be restricted in patients with pulmonary injury
(C) Blood transfusions should be considered in patients with PCV <30%
(D) Colloids are the recommended fluid for patients with brain injury

37. **Which of the following hormones is least likely to be a major influence on energy metabolism changes that occur in response to critical illness?**

(A) Glucagon
(B) Epinephrine
(C) Cortisol
(D) Insulin
(E) Thyroxine

38. **Critically ill animals lose weight even though they ingest food because:**

(A) Fat is burned in preference to carbohydrate
(B) Metabolic rate is invariably increased
(C) Cytokines cause enhanced muscle catabolism
(D) Malabsorption of nutrients from the gut occurs
(E) Ketogenesis requires significant ATP utilization

39. **Which of the following abnormalities is the hallmark of the refeeding syndrome?**

(A) Hypophosphatemia
(B) Hyperbilirubinemia
(C) Hyperammonemia
(D) Hypercholesterolemia
(E) Ketoacidosis

40. **Which of the following amino acids is crucial for maintenance of the GI mucosa?**

(A) Valine
(B) Leucine
(C) Taurine
(D) Glutamine
(E) Cysteine

41. **Calcium gluconate 10% should be used in patients in cardiopulmonary arrest who have which of the following**

(A) Hypokalemia
(B) Hyperkalemia
(C) Ventricular fibrillation
(D) Hypercalcemia

42. **Which of the following is the best cerebral-cardiopulmonary resuscitation technique for a 5-kg cat?**

(A) Dorsal recumbency, 80 compressions/min, manual ventilation at 10 breaths/min
(B) Lateral recumbency, 80 compressions/min, manual ventilation at 10 breaths/min
(C) Lateral recumbency, 120 compressions/min, manual ventilation at 30 breaths/min
(D) Dorsal recumbency, 120 compressions/min, manual ventilation at 20 breaths/min

43. **Which of the following cytokines is considered to be critical in the development of the systemic inflammatory response associated with sepsis?**

(A) IL-10
(B) PAF
(C) TNF
(D) IL-6
(E) IL-8

44. **Which of the following is considered to be an early clinical manifestation of sepsis?**

(A) Increased cardiac output
(B) Decreased pulmonary arterial pressure
(C) Increased systemic vascular resistance
(D) Decreased systemic arterial blood pressure
(E) Systemic arterial hypoxemia

45. **Which of the following antibiotic regimens would be best for empiric treatment of an animal with suspected sepsis?**

(A) Ampicillin and clindamycin
(B) Gentamicin and tetracycline
(C) Cefazolin and amikacin*
(D) Metronidazole and chloramphenicol
(E) Metronidazole and erythromycin

46. **Which of the following diagnostic test results is least likely to be observed in a septic patient?**

(A) Decreased serum lactate levels
(B) Elevated white blood cell count
(C) Decreased platelet count
(D) Hyperbilirubinemia
(E) Decreased blood glucose concentration

47. **Vitamin K–dependent factors are:**

(A) II, VIII, IX, XI
(B) II, IV, X, XII
(C) II, VII, IX, X
(D) II, III, IX, X

48. **Which of the follow statements is correct?**

(A) Factor XIa converts factor X to Xa
(B) A primary clot can be formed as long as there is a normal number of platelets
(C) All coagulation proteins are produced in the liver
(D) The major component in the fibrinolysis system is plasminogen

49. **Clinical signs of disseminated intravascular coagulation consist of:**

(A) Kidney failure
(B) Dyspnea
(C) Hemoabdomen
(D) All of the above

50. **Which of the following is diagnostic of disseminated intravascular coagulation?**

(A) Normal platelet count, low PT
(B) Elevated PT, elevated PTT, normal fibrinogen level, no FDPs
(C) Low platelet, low fibrinogen, normal PT and PTT, low AT III
(D) B and C

51. **Why are cats more sensitive to sodium nitroprusside administration than dogs?**

(A) It is difficult to get an IV catheter in cats
(B) Cyanide toxicity is more likely to occur in cats than dogs
(C) They are not more sensitive to nitroprusside administration
(D) You cannot measure blood pressure in cats and therefore monitoring of nitroprusside administration is impossible

52. **Signs of hypertension include:**

(A) Ataxia or seizures
(B) Epistaxis
(C) Acute blindness
(D) All of the above

53. **Treatment with which of the following classes of drugs may predispose an animal to hyperthermia from heatstroke?**

(A) Antibiotics
(B) Anticoagulants
(C) Diuretics
(D) Bronchodilators
(E) GI motility modifiers

54. **Which of the following organ system dysfunctions is most likely to occur following a severe hyperthermic event in a patient?**

(A) Congestive heart failure
(B) Acute renal failure
(C) Respiratory muscle paralysis
(D) Spinal cord dysfunction
(E) Adrenal insufficiency

55. **Which of the following is required for rewarming a severely hypothermic patient?**

(A) Wrapping in blankets
(B) Peritoneal lavage
(C) Heating pads
(D) Radiant heat lamps
(E) Submersion in a warm bath

56. **Which of the following laboratory abnormalities would most likely occur in a hypothermic patient?**

(A) Hemodilution
(B) Metabolic alkalosis
(C) Hyperlactatemia
(D) Hypernatremia
(E) Thrombocytosis

57. **Colonization of the GI tract by pathogenic bacteria is prevented by all of the following *except*:**

(A) Anaerobic enteric bacteria
(B) Gastric motility
(C) Prophylactic antibiotics
(D) Salivary flow
(E) Secretory IgA

58. **An antibiotic should *not***

(A) Be selected based on culture and sensitivity results
(B) Have a narrow spectrum of activity targeting the organisms suspected in a given infection
(C) Be given to prevent an infection when an invasive device (such as a urinary catheter) is placed
(D) Be used when there is evidence of existing infection

59. **What would be your first choice as treatment when presented with a dyspneic cat in shock?**

(A) IV catheter and bolus $1/2$ shock dose of fluids
(B) Thoracic radiographs
(C) A thorough physical examination and history
(D) Flow-by oxygen
(E) IV dexamethasone sodium phosphate

60. **Which one of the following is incorrect?**

(A) An animal is hypoxemic if the PaO_2 is <60 mm Hg
(B) Measurement of SpO_2 is a less accurate way to determine hypoxemia than SaO_2
(C) Acute respiratory distress syndrome is 1 example of diffusion impairment
(D) The 3 components of oxygen delivery are PaO_2, hemoglobin concentration, and heart rate
(E) A ventilation-perfusion mismatch can be caused by a pulmonary thromboembolism

61. **The most correct statement regarding inhibitory neuro-transmission is:**

(A) It involves membrane hyperpolarization of the neuron
(B) The predominant CNS neurotransmitter is glutamate
(C) It involves the influx of sodium and calcium
(D) It is most commonly increased with seizures

62. **The most incorrect statement regarding the treatment of seizures is:**

(A) Benzodiazepines given IV are an effective emergency anti-epileptic strategy
(B) The goal is to decrease depolarization or increase hyper-polarization of the cell
(C) Therapy is started when a structural brain lesion has been identified
(D) Status epilepticus with partial seizures need not be treated as an emergency

63. **All of the following are appropriate general treatment recommendations for patients with intracranial hyper-tension *except*:**

(A) Hyperventilation
(B) Mannitol
(C) Hypertonic saline solution
(D) Maintenance fluid therapy

64. **The cerebral ischemic response and Cushing's reflex in-clude:**

(A) Systemic hypertension and tachycardia
(B) Systemic hypertension and bradycardia
(C) Systemic hypotension and tachycardia
(D) Systemic hypotension and bradycardia

65. **Excessive activation of which of the following leads to the development of ischemic acute renal failure?**

(A) Prostaglandin synthesis
(B) Renin-angiotensin system
(C) Parasympathetic nerves
(D) Tubuloglomerular feedback
(E) Nitric oxide synthase

66. **The intracellular accumulation of which of the following is thought to be key to the development of cellular injury and death in ischemic acute renal failure?**

(A) Nitric oxide
(B) Prostaglandin E_2
(C) Calcium
(D) Ammonia
(E) Tumor necrosis factor

67. **Which of the following found by urine sediment examina-tion would suggest ethylene glycol poisoning in an animal with oliguria?**

(A) Oxalate crystals
(B) Urate crystals
(C) Triple phosphate crystals
(D) Struvite crystals
(E) Cystine crystals

68. **Which of the following best fits the electrolyte and acid-base findings expected in an animal with oliguric acute renal failure?**

(A) Metabolic acidosis, hypokalemia, hypernatremia
(B) Metabolic alkalosis, hyperkalemia, hypernatremia

(C) Metabolic alkalosis, hypokalemia, hyponatremia
(D) Metabolic acidosis, hyperkalemia, hypernatremia
(E) Metabolic alkalosis, normokalemia, normonatremia

69. **In oliguric acute renal failure, which of the following treatments can be used to induce increased urine pro-duction?**

(A) Dopamine
(B) Enalapril
(C) Prednisone
(D) Plasma
(E) Diltiazem

70. **Which of the following statements concerning peritoneal dialysis is most true?**

(A) Dialysate with 4% glucose concentration is the standard formulation commonly administered
(B) The usual volume of dialysate infused into the abdomen of the patient is 20 mL/kg
(C) In the uremic animal, dialysis is initiated with dialysate ex-changes every 4 hours
(D) Failure to retrieve 90% of the dialysate as effluent sug-gests a mechanical drainage problem
(E) Room-temperature dialysate is preferred for infusion into the peritoneal cavity

71. **Which of the following statements concerning congestive heart failure associated with primary diastolic dysfunc-tion is most correct?**

(A) It most commonly occurs in Doberman pinschers and cocker spaniels
(B) The most common clinical manifestation is ascites
(C) It is associated with increased left ventricular compliance
(D) It results in diminished activation of renin-angiotensin-aldo-sterone axis
(E) It results from concentric hypertrophy of the ventricular myocardium

72. **Which of the following catecholamines is preferred for use in the treatment of a patient with acute congestive heart failure and poor cardiac output?**

(A) Epinephrine
(B) Isoproterenol
(C) Norepinephrine
(D) Dobutamine
(E) Dopamine

73. **Which of the following would be the most important to consider in animals with sinus bradycardia?**

(A) Serum potassium concentration
(B) Packed cell volume
(C) Chest radiographs
(D) BUN concentration
(E) Thyroid hormone levels

74. **Which of the following statements is most true with re-spect to atrioventricular (AV) block?**

(A) First-degree AV block can be type I or type II
(B) Second-degree block results in dissociation of P and QRS complexes

(C) Second-degree block responds to cholinergic drug treatment
(D) Third-degree AV block requires pacemaker implantation
(E) First-degree AV block is often associated with syncope

75. **Which of the following antiarrhythmic drugs would be the empirical therapeutic choice for the treatment of atrial tachycardia in a dog with cardiomegaly?**

(A) Digoxin
(B) Lidocaine
(C) Propranolol
(D) Diltiazem
(E) Propantheline

76. **Ventricular fibrillation is treated by electrical defibrillation and the administration of which of the following drugs?**

(A) Lidocaine
(B) Digoxin
(C) Epinephrine
(D) Diltiazem
(E) Atropine

77. **Which of the following antibacterial agents is useful in diminishing ammonia-producing bacteria in the GI tract of animals with hepatic encephalopathy?**

(A) Clindamycin
(B) Metronidazole
(C) Ampicillin
(D) Tetracycline
(E) Chloramphenicol

78. **In animals with liver failure and ascites, which fluid crystalloid would you choose for initial empirical administration?**

(A) 0.9% Saline solution
(B) Lactated Ringer's solution
(C) 5% Dextrose in water
(D) Normosol-R
(E) 0.45% Saline and 2.5% dextrose

79. **Which of the following statements about acute pancreatitis is correct?**

(A) Most cases of acute pancreatitis in dogs and cats are caused by high-fat diets
(B) Common clinical signs in cats with acute pancreatitis include vomiting and abdominal pain
(C) Animals with severe acute pancreatitis may present with signs of shock, respiratory distress, bleeding dyscrasias, and oliguric renal failure
(D) Acute pancreatitis can be diagnosed definitively by laboratory testing

80. **Therapy for acute pancreatitis involves:**

(A) Surgical intervention for all severely affected animals
(B) Aggressive IV fluid therapy and anticipation of and early intervention against systemic complications
(C) Use of antibiotics for all affected animals
(D) Nutritional support for all affected animals

81. **Which of the following electrolyte and acid-base derangements is most likely to be observed during the diagnosis and treatment of diabetic ketoacidosis in a dog or cat?**

(A) Metabolic alkalosis
(B) Hypernatremia
(C) Hypokalemia
(D) Respiratory acidosis
(E) Hypochloremia

82. **Which of the following regimens is recommended for initial stabilization of the animal with diabetic ketoacidosis?**

(A) Regular insulin by intramuscular administration
(B) NPH insulin by intramuscular administration
(C) Ultra-lente insulin by constant-rate IV infusion
(D) Regular insulin by intermittent IV bolus administration
(E) NPH insulin by subcutaneous administration

Answers

1. **The answer is D.**

2. **The answer is D.**

3. **The answer is A.**

4. **The answer is C.**

5. **The answer is E.**

6. **The answer is B.**

7. **The answer is D.**

8. **The answer is B.**

9. **The answer is D.**

10. **The answer is B.**

11. **The answer is D.**

12. **The answer is B.**

13. **The answer is D.**

14. **The answer is D.**

15. **The answer is B.**
The primary disturbance is an acidosis because of the decreased pH. Since the HCO_3^- is not decreased from normal, the disturbance is not a primary metabolic one. Since the PCO_2 is increased from normal, the disturbance is a primary respiratory one. Based on the normal values listed, the expected compensatory response would be an increase in HCO_3^- above normal by 3.5 mmol/L in the acute situation. There is also a degree of hypoxemia present; thus, supplemental oxygen therapy may be beneficial.

16. **The answer is D.**
Since the pH is decreased, an acidosis is present. Evaluation of the PCO_2 leads to the expectation that a primary respiratory acidosis exists. Rules regarding compensation lead one to expect the HCO_3^- to be increased, which is not the case. Since the HCO_3^- is decreased with a decreased pH, a primary metabolic acidosis is also suspected. Since the PCO_2 and HCO_3^- are changing in opposite directions, a mixed acid-base disturbance is present.

17. **The answer is A.**
No hard and fast rules exist regarding when to treat metabolic acidosis. Cardiovascular complications from metabolic acidosis have been noted when the pH is <7.2 and the $[HCO_3^-]$ is <10 mEq/L. Adequate ventilation must be ensured prior to HCO_3^- administration since carbon dioxide is likely to be generated. Potential complications of $NaHCO_3$ administration include hypernatremia, hypokalemia, hypocalcemia, iatrogenic alkalosis, vascular volume overload, and paradoxical CSF acidosis. However, fear of complications should not take precedence over providing therapy for a potentially life-threatening condition.

18. **The answer is C.**
The acidosis and bicarbonate deficits are severe enough to warrant $NaHCO_3$ replacement therapy. Based on the equation given in Chapter 9 (assuming normal $HCO_3^- = 20$ mEq/L), there is an HCO_3^- deficit of 66 mEq. To administer $NaHCO_3$, first ensure that the patient is able to ventilate adequately. Then administer half of the deficit (33 mEq $NaHCO_3$) IV over 2–3 hours. Following the infusion, blood gas values and electrolyte levels should be rechecked to see if further bicarbonate therapy is needed and to see if there are any electrolyte derangements that need to be corrected.

19. **The answer is A.**
Aspirin toxicity can lead to a metabolic acidosis and a respiratory alkalosis. A pyothorax leads to hypoventilation by preventing the lungs from fully expanding, morphine leads to hypoventilation through CNS-mediated effects, and fluid overload can lead to pulmonary edema, which affects gas exchange by increasing the diffusion barrier or the V/Q mismatch.

20. **The answer is C.**
With chronic respiratory acidosis, aggressive supplemental oxygen therapy is not warranted as hypoxemia may be what is driving the patient to ventilate. At the same time, aggressive ventilator therapy is not necessarily warranted because the disease is likely chronic in nature, and once the patient is removed from ventilator support, the PCO_2 will likely increase again. Bicarbonate therapy is not indicated because this is a problem of ventilation, and supplemental $NaHCO_3$ will increase the generation of carbon dioxide, which the patient is already having difficulty eliminating. The proper therapy of chronic respiratory acidosis is fluids with adequate Cl^-. The Cl^- allows the kidneys to excrete the excess HCO_3^- the body has been retaining as compensation.

21. **The answer is D.**
Removal of the gastric foreign body resolves the underlying cause of the metabolic alkalosis. However, the maintenance factors of volume depletion, hypokalemia, and increased aldosterone secretion are present. The provision of adequate volumes of chloride-containing fluids with adequate potassium supplementation will help eliminate these maintenance factors.

22. **The answer is B.**
Treatment should be aimed at correcting the underlying disorder, in this case, hypoxemia. Hypocapnia in itself is not a major threat to the well-being of the patient in this instance.

23. **The answer is D.**
Blood passing through an intracardiac or intrapulmonary right-to-left shunt will not contact alveoli to allow diffusion of oxygen into the blood.

24. **The answer is A.**

25. **The answer is D.**

26. **The answer is C.**

27. **The answers are A, B, and D.**

28. The answer is D.

29. The answer is C.
General anesthesia prevents pain perception during surgery but does not limit nociceptive input to the spinal cord and higher centers. Nociceptive input sensitizes the nociceptors, peripheral neurons, and CNS to painful impulses. Therefore, postoperative pain is not diminished by the use of general anesthesia alone.

30. The answer is F.
Epidural analgesia can reduce the requirements for general anesthetics and thus is useful in patients with hepatic disease and reduced drug clearance and in patients with renal disease in whom the potential hypotension during anesthesia may decrease renal perfusion. A reduction in depth of anesthesia may help to maintain pulmonary function in patients with pulmonary contusions and to prevent the need for manual ventilation, which may rupture pulmonary bullae. Epidural analgesics should not be administered if there is lumbosacral trauma or if there are contaminated wounds or skin infections that could lead to the introduction of bacteria into the epidural space.

31. The answer is E.

32. The answer is B.

33. The answer is B.

34. The answer is B.

35. The answer is E.

36. The answer is C.

37. The answer is E.

38. The answer is C.

39. The answer is A.

40. The answer is D.

41. The answer is B.

42. The answer is C.

43. The answer is C.

44. The answer is A.

45. The answer is C.

46. The answer is A.

47. The answer is C.

48. The answer is D.
Factor XIa converts factor IX to IXa, not Xa. A primary clot *cannot* be formed if there is a platelet dysfunction disorder. Factor VIII is produced by vascular endothelial cells and megakaryocytes, not by the liver.

49. The answer is D.
Kidney failure can occur if a thrombus is located in the renal artery; dyspnea, if pulmonary thromboemboli are present; and hemoabdomen, if there is a complete consumption of coagulation factors.

50. The answer is C.
A is not correct because of the normal platelet count. B is not correct because the fibrinogen level should be low with an elevated PT and PTT if disseminated intravascular coagulation is occurring. This might be a warfarin-type toxicity.

51. The answer is B.
Cyanide toxicity is more likely to occur in cats than dogs because of cats' reduced ability to conjugate cyanide to thiocyanate in the liver. The kidney removes thiocyanate from circulation, so animals with renal insufficiency are also at risk for cyanide toxicity.

52. The answer is D.
Animals presenting with hypertension often have a history of ataxia or seizures, epistaxis, or acute blindness due to the end-organ effects of acute, severe hypertension.

53. The answer is C.

54. The answer is B.

55. The answer is B.

56. The answer is C.

57. The answer is C.
The use of antibiotics can decrease or alter the populations of normal enteric bacteria that play a role in preventing the adhesion and multiplication of new organisms.

58. The answer is C.
Antibiotics should be used rarely to prevent infection. When an invasive device is placed, the site and the patient should be monitored for signs of infection. If infection is detected, the device should be removed if possible, and antibiotic therapy started. The use of antibiotics prior to the development of infection increases the risk of infection with resistant bacteria and contributes to the selection pressure exerted on environmental bacteria, increasing the likelihood that resistance will develop.

59. The answer is D.
The quickest and most beneficial treatment is to provide oxygen. Then the patient's history can be obtained while a physical examination is performed.

60. The answer is D.
The 3 components of oxygen delivery are PaO_2, hemoglobin concentration, and cardiac output. Cardiac output is equal to the heart rate times the stroke volume.

61. The answer is A.

62. The answer is D.

63. The answer is A.

64. The answer is B.

65. **The answer is B.**

66. **The answer is C.**

67. **The answer is A.**

68. **The answer is D.**

69. **The answer is A.**

70. **The answer is D.**

71. **The answer is E.**

72. **The answer is D.**

73. **The answer is A.**

74. **The answer is D.**

75. **The answer is A.**

76. **The answer is C.**

77. **The answer is B.**

78. **The answer is E.**

79. **The answer is C.**

80. **The answer is B.**

81. **The answer is C.**

82. **The answer is A.**

References

Boldt J, et al. Influence of different volume therapies on circulating soluble adhesion molecules in critically ill patients. Crit Care Med 24:385–391, 1996.

DiBartola S. Disorders of potassium: Hypokalemia and hyperkalemia. In: Fluid therapy in small animal practice. Philadelphia: WB Saunders, 1992; Pp. 89–115.

Drummond JC, et al. The effect of the reduction of colloid oncotic pressure on post-traumatic cerebral edema. Anesthesiology 88:993–1002, 1998.

Hendrix PK, Raffe MR, et al. Epidural administration of bupivicaine, morphine, or their combination for postoperative analgesia in dogs. JAVMA 209:598–607, 1996.

Jenkins WL. Pharmacologic aspects of analgesic drugs in animals: an overview. JAVMA 191:1231–1240, 1987.

King LG. Colloid osmometry: Curr Vet Ther XIII in Bonagura JD (ed). p 116–118, 2000.

Mathews KA. Nonsteroidal anti-inflammatory analgesics in pain management in dogs and cats. Can Vet J 37:539–545, 1996.

Morisaki H, et al. Compared with crystalloid, colloid therapy slows progression of extrapulmonary tissue injury in septic sheep. J Appl Physiol 25:1507–1518, 1997.

Nelson LD, et al. New advances in the care of critically injured patients. New Horizons 7:1–172, 1999.

Nielson VG, et al. Hetastarch solution decreases multiple organ injury and xanthine oxidase release after hepatoenteric ischemia-reperfusion in rabbits. Crit Care Med 25:1565–1574, 1997.

Phillips SL, Polzin DJ. Clinical disorders of potassium homeostasis. Vet Clin North Am 28:545–564, 1998.

Quandt JE, Rawlings CR. Reducing postoperative pain for dogs: Local anesthetic and analgesic techniques. Compendium 18:101–111, 1996.

Short CE, Poznak AV. Animal pain. New York: Churchill Livingstone, 1992.

T-L Choi P, et al. Crystalloids versus colloids in fluid resuscitation; a systematic review. Crit Care Med 27:200–210, 1999.

Willard MD. Disorders of potassium homeostasis. Vet Clin North Am 19:241–263, 1989.

Index